Dr. Gyl's Guide

to a Successful
Hearing Care Practice

Editor-in-Chief for Audiology
Brad A. Stach, PhD

Dr. Gyl's Guide

to a Successful Hearing Care Practice

Gyl Kasewurm, AuD

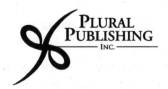

PLURAL
PUBLISHING
INC.

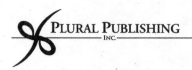

5521 Ruffin Road
San Diego, CA 92123

e-mail: information@pluralpublishing.com
Website: https://www.pluralpublishing.com

Typeset in 11/13 Garamond by Flanagan's Publishing Services, Inc.
Printed in the United States of America by Integrated Books International
21 20 19   2 3 4 5

Library of Congress Cataloging-in-Publication Data

Names: Kasewurm, Gyl A., author.
Title: Dr. Gyl's guide to a successful hearing care practice / Gyl Kasewurm.
Other titles: Guide to a successful hearing care practice
Description: San Diego, CA : Plural Publishing, [2019] | Includes
   bibliographical references and index.
Identifiers: LCCN 2018055068| ISBN 9781635502077 (alk. paper) | ISBN
   1635502071 (alk. paper)
Subjects: | MESH: Audiology | Practice Management—standards | Private
   Practice—organization & administration | Private Practice—economics |
   Marketing of Health Services
Classification: LCC RF291 | NLM WV 21 | DDC 617.80068—dc23
LC record available at https://lccn.loc.gov/2018055068

Contents

Contents

Preface

> You Become What You Believe You Are.
> Change Your Thoughts and You Change
> Your World.

This guide is a collection of business and life lessons I have found to be valuable throughout my career as a business owner. It is also a compilation of many articles I have written over the years. It is dedicated to anyone who dreams of becoming an entrepreneur and building a happy, successful, and rewarding life as a business owner, and also to all the practice managers who continually search for new ways to build a stronger and more profitable practice.

—Dr. Gyl

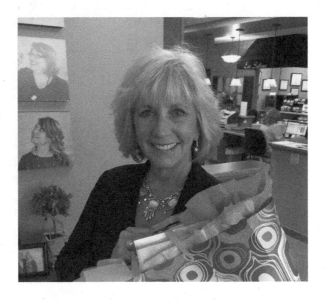

Purpose of the Guide

My degree in audiology neither taught nor prepared me to operate a successful business. I have faced many challenges over the past thirty plus years as a business owner. When faced with difficulties, I have sought advice from the best and brightest professionals in hopes they could help teach me how to create and sustain a profitable practice. What I have learned is that business is business, no matter what type of business you are in. This guide will focus on ways to assess the health of a business and explain how to make a few, simple changes that can have a dramatic impact on the profitability and productivity of a practice.

Owning and operating your own business can, and most certainly will, be fraught with obstacles and challenges. Most hearing health care practices employ one professional and one support person, which usually means that the hearing professional spends the majority of her or his time seeing patients, and then has to find some additional time to complete the tasks that are required to insure the business run smoothly. Consequently, the owner can't always devote, or doesn't want to devote their "free time," to make certain the business is as profitable or efficient as it could be.

For many years, hearing health care professionals have had the luxury of being in a high margin, low volume business. Consequently, most practices have been able to survive despite a lack of attention to key performance indicators of the business. Sustainability in this economy is commendable, but imagine increasing profits by as much as 50% or more while operating the same business and doing only a slightly better job. It doesn't take many changes to accomplish just that. This guide highlights some of the easiest ways to improve the profitability of a practice.

I recall an article written by my colleague, practice management expert Brian Taylor, which reported the results of an investigation into the business practices of a small group of hearing health care providers. His investigation revealed that the average practitioner thought their business was doing much better than it actually was. Self-impressions can be inaccurate, but numbers tell the real story of how well a business is doing. Once you know the facts, implementing just a few simple changes can substantially increase profitability.

One thing is certain—the business of health care is changing and hearing health care is no exception. Most hearing health care practices have depended on the sale of hearing aids to generate the majority of gross revenue for the business. In today's market, consumers can literally go anywhere to purchase hearing aids, even to a low-cost wholesaler, not to mention the endless opportunities to purchase hearing aids on the internet. In addition to many purchasing options, insurance companies are cutting reimbursements, eliminating coverage for hearing health care services, and promoting discount programs to their subscribers ,which usually further reduces revenue for private practitioners. Furthermore, most hearing aid manufacturers have increased their presence in the retail market. Although these observations may cause concern, I am reminded that with obstacles come opportunities. However, to maximize opportunities, you must be prepared and willing to modify and/or change the way you conduct business. If you notice that your bottom line is shrinking but are unsure how to assess what the problem might be, this guide may be just what you need to determine the health of the practice, and will hopefully provide ideas on how to infuse new energy and life into the business.

In today's tough, economic climate, even experienced practice owners can't rely on what worked in the past to guarantee success in the future, and must continually monitor the health of the business and search for ways to improve and to maximize profitability. I hope this guide will help readers do just that!

1
Getting Started in Private Practice

I am often asked what it takes to start a private practice. Married and living in a small town with no hope of local employment, I started my practice immediately following graduation from graduate school because I didn't feel I had much choice if I wanted to work as an audiologist. What I lacked in experience I made up for in ambition. I have experienced numerous highs and lows throughout my career, but I have never regretted the decision to start my own practice. Although technology, management styles, hearing aid distribution, and the economy have changed, the necessary requirements of being an entrepreneur remain the same today as they were many years ago when I started my business: keep an eye on the key indicators of profitability, market to the general public and current patients, keep your referral sources close, adhere to best practices, and hold any and all employees accountable for doing their jobs.

Starting and sustaining a business takes the same level of commitment and desire it takes to maintain a successful relationship. If you want your business to be successful, you are going to have to work at it and make it a top priority. Once you decide to start a practice and set the wheels in motion, there is no looking back—only ahead. If you do things right, the future can be very bright and profitable.

Step One

The first step in starting a business is to develop a good plan that will serve as a solid foundation for the practice. Writing a business plan is the best way to gauge whether or not *your* business is viable for *your* marketplace. The business plan will become the blueprint for the practice and the driving force for many years to come. Most contractors wouldn't start building a new home without first having a good house plan, and starting a business without a business plan would be just as foolish.

Although having a well-written and thought-out business plan is an essential first step in starting a practice, you will also need enough working capital to cover operating expenses and your salary for at least the first six months of operation, and preferably a year. The business plan will serve as the foundation for obtaining possible funding for the venture.

It is also paramount that you are a top-notch, knowledgeable, hearing health care professional who possesses solid, technical skills to provide the highest quality of care in diagnosing and treating hearing problems. The aspects of business you don't know you can learn. You can also hire people to teach you the things you don't understand, but your professional expertise is what will attract and keep patients. Whereas business and professional skills are important, an entrepreneur must possess the internal fortitude to know success *can* and *will* happen. When times get tough, you may reflect, but you must focus on existing or future opportunities. I once read that good entrepreneurs have their feet firmly planted on the ground, their hearts in the business, and their heads in the clouds. If you don't believe that opportunity exists and you have what it takes to uncover it, you may not survive the hard times that are sure to come along in the life of a business. My father used to say he never saw anyone who could be as stubborn as I could be. That quality has proven to be invaluable for me over the years.

> When things aren't going well, think about what you CAN do and not about what you CAN'T do. Every obstacle can become an opportunity.

Although there are many advantages to owning your own business, in the beginning you will have to be prepared to sacrifice things such as paid vacations, and perhaps, even necessities, like a salary. Being an entrepreneur involves taking a risk and operating without the safety net that salaried employees are used to, such as paid insurance coverage, PTO for holidays and vacations, and funded pension plans, but if you persist and the business becomes profitable, you will realize many more benefits than any employee ever will.

Before starting a practice, you should ask yourself if you like being in charge and enjoy making decisions. If you don't, private practice may not be for you. Successful business owners are continually forced to make snap decisions and must live with the results of those decisions. Being the decision maker is actually one of the aspects of owning a business that inspires many entrepreneurs, but some people just don't have the internal fortitude to handle such responsibility. It's a good idea to explore how you feel about this aspect of entrepreneurship before you enter into business. The website, http://www.Entrepreneur.com, has many good articles and assessments that may help you assess the feasibility of starting your own business and whether your personality style lends itself to being an entrepreneur.

An insatiable drive alone is not enough to start and maintain a successful business. You must also have the discipline and determination to weather the storms that will come, and the endurance to do whatever it takes to survive and thrive after the storms. Successful business people are tenacious; obstacles simply represent temporary barriers to overcome on the road to greater opportunities. They may take "no" for an answer, but only for as long as it takes to reframe the question from another perspective.

Having a good support system is helpful when you start a new business. I would recommend that a neophyte find an experienced practitioner to serve as a mentor during the early years of business. Whereas going it alone and running the show may sound attractive, being a business owner can be a lonely road, especially during the early years of a business. It is very helpful to have someone to bounce ideas off of when faced with the uncertainty of a major decision. It's no coincidence that many successful small business owners have some type of partner, whether it's a business partner or a life partner. I could never have succeeded in practice all these years without the tireless and unconditional support of my husband. Although he questions some of my crazy ideas, and that can be a good thing, he is my biggest advocate when the ideas are implemented (Figure 1–1).

When you own your own business, you are the person who is ultimately in control of everything. Although that can be empowering, it also means that the buck stops with YOU. At the end of the day, it will be up to you, the business owner or practice manager, to solve problems and to make sure the business succeeds. Some people start their own practice because they are tired of being at the mercy of a boss, but a business owner is at the mercy of the business. An owner is able to control their schedule and have the flexibility to work around family or personal obligations, but may also have to work more than 40 hours a week to get the job done. On the flip side, an owner will never have to ask permission to take a vacation or to take a day off.

For some people, owning a business is part of the American Dream, not to mention that it can offer increased earning potential and many tax advantages. A business owner can write off items that employees can't. However, being the business owner means you must be prepared to give up the security of a regular

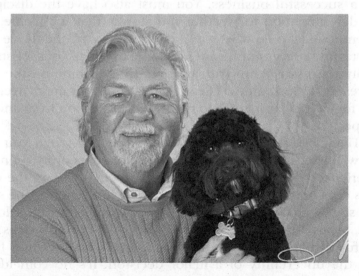

Figure 1–1. My husband, David, and our fur baby, Eddie.

paycheck. You will never have to ask the boss for a raise, but you may not be able to afford to give yourself one. If you think you can handle this sort of uncertainty, that's good, because be assured that a business owner is faced with uncertainty on a daily basis. Business owners are rarely faced with boredom because they are so busy wearing many different hats, which may include marketing wizard, HR manager, bookkeeper, IT director, secretary, and president all rolled into one. However, when you are the boss, you have the independence to create your own policies and procedures. You won't have to ask anyone's approval when you want to create a new policy or redecorate the office. You can do things *your* way. You literally have the opportunity to create the practice of your dreams, but sometimes, dreams can come with an occasional nightmare.

In the beginning, you may not be able to afford to hire an employee, but as the business grows, you will certainly be faced with the job of managing, training, and motivating employees, a job for which most hearing health care professionals have little or no training. You may end up spending a lot of time attending to the details of running a business and less time on things you really enjoy doing, such as playing golf, coaching your kids' sports, or entertaining. It's not uncommon as a business owner to be forced to undertake tasks you find unpleasant, such as firing someone or refusing to hire a friend or relative. Employee management continues to be a challenge for me. I like to believe that a person will just "do their job" but that is not usually the case. Employees need to be managed and held accountable for the tasks they are responsible for, and when they aren't held accountable, performance is certain to slide, and that will most definitely affect business. When you start a practice, you have the opportunity to gain experience in every facet of business, and when the business succeeds, you will have the unparalleled joy of knowing your management and direction were responsible for that success.

Entrepreneurs often have many traits in common; chief among them is a willingness to take a risk. Not a blind risk, but a calculated, prudent risk for which you must be prepared. If you are considering venturing into private practice, it is crucial to take some business courses and find a good mentor who will agree to guide you in the beginning. I have found that a good

CPA and a knowledgeable attorney are vital advisors to a business owner, and even seasoned business owners have to periodically seek advice on how to improve business.

I don't have to spend much time wondering whether owning a practice has been the right choice for me. It has been and continues to be fun and exciting, but I have faced enough challenges over the years to know it's not the right choice for everyone.

Timeline for a New Practice

Twelve Months Prior to Opening

- Determine whether starting a practice is the best opportunity
- Begin developing a business plan
- Assess competition
- Explore possible geographical locations
- Investigate financing options
  - Conventional loan versus SBA loan
  - Manufacturer loan
- Establish budget for the project
- View commercial real estate properties in desired area
- Gather quotes for building-out potential offices spaces
- Compile quotes for equipment
- Determine opening date for the practice

Eight Months Prior to Opening

- Meet with community resources
- Determine insurance needs
- Meet with at least two marketing groups for ideas and quotes for services

- o Determine marketing materials that are needed
- Apply for state licensure if necessary

Six Months Prior to Opening

- Consult with attorney and CPA to determine the most appropriate entity of business
- Have professional photos taken
- EMR software: compare available options
  - o (visit http://www.audiologysoftware.com to compare)
- Determine best location and sign lease on property
- Meet with architect to design floor plan
- Meet with bank regarding loan
- Meet with equipment representative to review specifications and questions. Ask about start-up discounts, installation, and training
- Create marketing plan for first six months of operation
- Choose logo design
- Obtain insurance for professional liability and business
  - o Professional liability insurance through one of the professional associations is much more affordable than through private entity

Four Months Prior to Opening

- Have promotional items available: business cards, brochures
- Develop pricing for services and products
- Create protocols and develop necessary forms
- Apply for NPIs
- Start process for any insurance credentialing
- Open bank accounts
- Start construction for build-out

- Order equipment
- Order furniture
- Order exterior signs for building
- Develop website
- Meet with radio and television stations regarding advertising and demographics

Three Months Prior to Opening

- Submit credit applications to manufacturers
- Meet with IT—choose and order computers, router, monitors, flat screens, speakers, printers, and so forth
- Establish e-mail addresses
- Select a business telephone system
- Advertise opening date
- Apply for state sales tax license

One Month Prior to Opening

- Publish press releases
- Delivery of furniture, computers
- Order audiology supplies
- Purchase office supplies
- Install Internet and telephone
- Install audiology equipment and learn how to use

2

A Plan to Build On

Earlier in this guide, I suggested that if you want to open a practice, the first step is to create a well-written business plan. I have read the sentiment that "those who fail to plan, plan to fail" and in my opinion there is nothing truer when it comes to business. It's similar to inviting friends to a fancy dinner party and then not making any specific plans to insure the party will be a success. It's important to try to control your own destiny, and in business that means having specific plans, roadmaps, and budgets that serve as guides when making day-to-day business decisions. A good plan should define a set of goals and should outline the actions necessary to achieve those goals. However, a plan must also include the flexibility for intervention when something isn't working or when unexpected disruptions in the market necessitate change. The plan should be fluid and open to change. Sometimes, you can pound a market that isn't working and exhaust your budget. It's like trying to fit a round peg into a square hole, and of course, that just won't work.

Lego Corporation originally started their business by making wooden ducks. A few years later after a fire burned down the factory, management decided to switch to making plastic toys and the resultant interlocking bricks spawned a multibillion-dollar business. They could have persevered on their original course with disastrous outcomes but they had the foresight to see when change was necessary.

Although most people go into business with the *hope* that things will work out, and the belief that they will do everything they can to make the business succeed, careful planning and a thought-out business plan are the foundation of successful businesses. Business planning is the process of creating a model or envisioning a picture of your goals and expectations for the business. Business plans are inherently strategic. You start *here* today with certain resources and abilities, and you know you want to get to *there*, a point in the future (usually three to five years out), at which time your business will have a different set of resources and abilities, as well as greater profitability and increased assets. The purpose of the plan is to show how you will get from here to there. The business planning process is one of discovery and learning. It is a disciplined approach in which you ask questions, seek answers, and plan for the future of the business. A business plan describes who, what, when, where, why, and how of a good story. Although a business plan must present the facts, it should also stress your unique qualifications as the owner, and the impact that those qualities will have on the business and its potential customers. In other words, a good business plan should outline the structure of the business, forecast the bright future you have planned, and provide an inspiring story that will captivate and convince readers as to why the business will certainly be a success.

Business plans must include several elements that shouldn't be modified. Readers of the plan will expect to see a certain format and, especially in the case of financial backers, they may not take the plan seriously if they don't see those essential elements in the plan. A well-written plan has five fundamental components:

1. **Executive Summary**
2. **Business Section**
3. **Market Analysis**
4. **Financing Options**
5. **Management Section**

The business plan is a multipurpose tool containing several different sections that will assist the writer in planning and operating the business. Although the business plans of major corporations can stretch to several hundred pages, many entrepreneurs' plans may be as short as five pages. The length of each section should be tailored to the particular needs of the individual business owner and the information needed to convince readers that the business will succeed. Detailed planning may require consulting a fellow business person or hiring a consultant to examine every aspect of the organization before undertaking the necessary financial investment to make the enterprise happen. It is easy to change strategies, target markets, or the nature of the business on paper without losing any of your hard-earned or borrowed cash in real life.

The strategic portion of the business plan will serve as the heart of the document and should cover in detail your expectations for the first 12 months of the business, and outline the next two to five years in lesser detail. This phase investigates the business environment, the organization's capabilities, the competitive advantage, and the predicted basis for continued growth. The action steps should outline the primary objectives for the initial months in business and can also involve developing strategies for areas of the business that will be essential for profitability, such as cost of goods, charges of diagnostics, and reimbursement schedules.

In addition to probing possible strengths and weaknesses of the practice, the plan should paint a realistic view of the expectations and long-term objectives of the business. It is better to abandon an idea in its infancy than to invest a lot of time and money before learning that the idea will not work. For instance, most practitioners would agree that it is very difficult, and perhaps impossible, to sustain a practice on diagnostics alone, and it will be necessary to dispense hearing aids to maintain a profitable practice, especially in light of continual reductions in reimbursement and interference from third-party payers.

The executive summary is a very important part of the business plan. This brief statement, also known as the statement of purpose, addresses and explains key elements of the business and your objectives for starting it. If you are presenting the plan to financiers, the key synopsis of the business must capture their attention and convince them of the viability of the proposed plan. The executive summary is a quick overview of all aspects of the business in an attempt to introduce the proposed company to the readers (Figure 2–1).

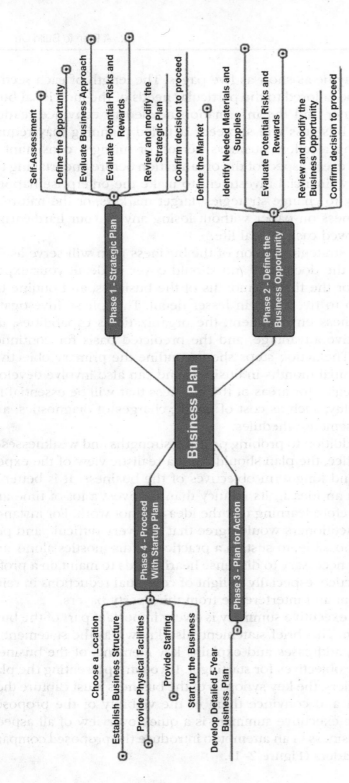

Figure 2–1. Sample organizational chart for a business plan.

If someone were to read only the executive summary—and many readers will never read past this point—he or she would learn the name and nature of the business, its legal structure, the amount of the loan request, and a repayment schedule. This is why your first statement must be convincing as to why the business is sure to succeed. Because this section introduces and summarizes the essence of the business plan, you must determine what you want the reader to know about your potential business, and it must be condensed into a few paragraphs that can be read and absorbed quickly and easily.

After completing the business plan, you will have a much better idea of what your practice will look like: the services that you will offer, the products you will dispense, your ideal patient, your biggest competition, the types and costs of marketing, the potential risks, and what kind of financing you will need to get started. The process of writing a business plan will help you identify whether your idea has potential for success and whether it is an idea worth pursuing. I know many of you may be wondering how you will have time to undertake what may seem an overwhelming task of developing a plan. Creating such a plan doesn't have to take a great deal of time if you have some performance goals in mind. There are many Internet resources available to help you do that, such as (http://www.sba.gov/tools/business-plan). Start with an outline and then develop an action plan of how you plan to reach those goals. A plan without specific goals is no more than wishful thinking. Business planning shouldn't just be a part of the early stages of a business. In fact, business owners should take the time to sit down and do a little planning at the beginning of each year, just to make sure that the new year will be a good one for business. Many practice owners are so busy working in their businesses that they don't take the time to create a formal, written plan for every new year. Our industry is inundated with new obstacles and hurdles that arise, so a formal plan with established goals can help ensure the business is on the right track. Wishing and hoping that business will go well really isn't enough in today's competitive and challenging environment. It really doesn't matter if the business is a start-up, or thirty years old, a written business plan is necessary to keep the business on track. Once you have written the plan and put it into place, it's a good idea to review it every three months to see what is working, what needs to be changed, and what fac-tors have affected the change. The business may be doing so well that it's necessary to accelerate the goals to more closely align with what is actually happening in the business. Don't get lulled into an "all or nothing" mentality. Creating and maintain-ing a successful business is about consistency and momentum. Visions can come and go, but if they are created with a clear and well-defined road map, success is more likely.

Goals Drive Success

Imagine having to shoot an arrow without being given a target. Where would you aim? And say you did aim at some random thing (out of sheer perplexity). Why would you aim there? And what would the purpose be? Get the idea? This is a literal exam-ple of what life is like without a goal or target in mind. It's point-less and a waste of energy and effort.

In my practice, we set monthly goals for each employee. For instance, goals for our professionals include, the number of hearing aid units sold, return for credit rate, patient satisfaction as determined by the surveys we send to patients and, of course, everyone is expected to adhere to best practices as determined by a needs study and verification of hearing aid benefit using real ear measurements and aided discrimination. Goals for sup-port personnel include, revenue generated as a result of services and repairs performed on hearing aids, and the responsibility of referring unhappy or dissatisfied patients back to their original professional for follow-up. In addition, satisfaction surveys are sent to patients that have been seen by our service department to ensure that patients are receiving the exceptional service that the business is known for.

Our goals are set to help push the business to new levels of success. We can't always count on the business going well, so we take steps to make certain things go well. You can have all the potential in the world but without focus, abilities, and talent are useless. Just like how sunlight can't burn through anything without a magnifying glass focusing it, you can't achieve any-thing unless a goal is focusing your effort. At the end of the day, goals are what give people and businesses direction. This sense of direction is what allows one's mind to focus on and hit a target rather than shooting aimlessly and wasting energy.

Most people spend more time planning their vacations than planning their lives. If you asked my husband about his golf vacation, he would tell you every explicit detail about the trip, but if you ask him when he is going to retire he will reply, "I don't know. I haven't really thought about it." I know many people like my husband who drift along in life without actually knowing where they want to go. They work hard but have no particular destination in mind. That may be an acceptable way to get through life, but history has shown that goal setters accomplish twice as much as those who don't. Although my husband reminds me that life isn't all about "accomplishing things," I have found that setting goals has definitely helped me drive my practice. There is no way that we could have produced millions in gross revenue in a small town without having very specific goals. If you don't know where you are going, chances are you may wander aimlessly without ever reaching your destination.

A key reason many people don't set goals is that they don't spend enough time thinking about what they really want out of life. Goal setting can serve as a powerful process for thinking about your ideal future, and for motivating yourself to turn your vision of this future into reality. By knowing precisely what you want to achieve, you know where to concentrate your efforts. You'll also quickly spot the distractions that can easily lead you off on a tangent that wastes time and money.

At its simplest, a goal is just a target to aim for, but goals can also be powerful motivators that contribute to personal or professional growth. The process of goal setting can force us to think through our desires and motivate us to work harder to get what we really want out of life. The key to goal setting is that the goals should be specific and measurable. Of course, it's nice to reach a goal, and some people have a tendency to set a goal very low so they know they can achieve it. There is nothing wrong with shooting for the stars. My mother used to say that I was the girl who wanted it all! She was right, and I always believed that any star was reachable if you worked hard enough and believed you could get there.

> If you dream it, you can achieve it.

Goal setting is important when it comes to business. Of course, the goal of any business is to be profitable. Most hearing health care professionals in private practice have lots of jobs to do, and it's easy to get overwhelmed and lose sight of the key aspects that contribute to profitability. This has happened to me many times. My written goals helped me get back on track. At the end of each month, I review my numbers and compare where I wanted to be with where I am. If business is off track, I dig in and determine where we are falling short of our goals and what we need to do differently to reach our goals.

We all have things that we want to achieve in our lives. Perhaps it's getting into better shape, building a successful business, raising a wonderful family, writing a best-selling book, or winning a sports challenge. Personally, I enjoy setting goals because I like working for something specific and I delight in the sense of accomplishment when I reach what may have initially seemed unattainable. We can *let* life happen, or we can *make* life happen. I prefer the latter.

> "If you aim at nothing, you will hit it every time."
> —Zig Ziglar

By setting goals, you give yourself mental boundaries. When you have a certain end point in mind, it's easier to avoid distractions and to stay focused toward accomplishing the goal. To get a better idea, imagine this. Your best friend is moving to Switzerland and his flight takes off at 9:00 PM. You leave right after work at 8:30 PM to see him off and you know it's a 20-minute walk to get to the airport. So you make it a goal to reach the airport in 15 minutes by jogging so that you can have more time to say your goodbyes. Would you get distracted by "anything" along the way? Would you stop for a break or a snack? Would you stop by your house before going to the airport? Probably not.

One-half of knowing what you want, is knowing what steps you will have to take to get it. By making a goal, you give yourself a concrete endpoint to aim for and something specific that you are working towards. A specific and SMART (Specific, Measureable, Assignable, Relevant, and Time-Based) goal can give direction to a business. A SMART goal can give a business owner or manager something very tangible to focus on, and helps explain to everyone in the organization exactly what they have to do to accomplish that goal. Setting goals is not a complicated process, nor does it take a lot of time, but "You have to set them to get them." Although setting goals is definitely easier than reaching them, top-performing businesses are driven by the very specific goals they set. Many businesses survive but never thrive because they fail to establish road maps in the form of goals to guide them.

To be effective, every goal should produce some sort of quantifiable result. For example, "I will increase total gross sales by 15% this year" is a measurable goal. The more specific the goal, the easier it is to accomplish. "I will start a private practice in Chicago before 2025" is a much more compelling goal than "I want to go into business for myself."

An important element of goal setting is to include deadlines. A goal without a deadline is simply a dream, and dreams don't always become a reality. Attach a realistic, yet challenging, deadline for an accomplishment and post it where you can review it regularly.

One of the most important steps for setting effective goals is quality over quantity. If you are not in the habit of setting goals, start with one or two realistic ones that will be easy to accomplish. You will start to build momentum once you see that you really can achieve your dreams when you put them in writing and have a realistic plan to accomplish them.

When setting goals, you have to remember that anything is possible, and you have to maintain a positive attitude. Don't say, "I want to." Say, "I will." The fact is most of us don't achieve our goals because we really don't believe we can. There is something to be said for the power of positive thinking. Instead of focusing on the negative, replace criticism you give to yourself with encouragement. Compliment yourself and those around you on what you have all achieved. The size of your success is determined by the size of your belief. Therefore, if you believe big, you will achieve big.

I have had many experiences when goals have pushed everyone in the practice to achieve greater success. I recall looking at the numbers in early December of 2010, and the three million dollar mark was in site, but a stretch to reach before the end of the year. When I reviewed the scheduled appointments, I really thought we would fall short, especially since the holidays were coming and several staff members were going to be off on vacation. I called the staff together and told them how close we were to reaching a HUGE goal, and added an extra incentive if we topped that three million dollar mark. I praised them for being a phenomenal team and assured them that while the goal may seem impossible, I truly believed that we could make it happen if we worked together. At 4:30 PM on December 31, with no more patients on the schedule, we were $3800 from the goal. The disappointment was tangible, but I told them not to give up. We still had 30 minutes!! The phone rang at 4:48 PM and a patient that had been seen earlier in the week decided to go ahead with an order for new aids! The $3995 sale put us over the mark! Never give up.

It is essential to monitor goals regularly to keep them foremost in your mind and to give a sense of how close you are to accomplishing them. If your business goals depend on employees, involve them so that everyone understands their particular role in achieving the goals. Once you've set the goals, schedule periodic progress meetings to keep everyone focused on the specific target. Positive feedback can make the difference between a goal that is accomplished and one that is missed by just a fraction.

I find that it's a motivator to reward yourself when you reach your goals: What will you or your business receive once your goals have been met? A bonus, a day off, a staff outing? Perhaps the reward is simply the satisfaction of knowing you accomplished your goals. Personal satisfaction is important, but sustained hard work and effort should lead to more tangible rewards as well.

Goals help push individuals and organizations to greater heights, and you will be amazed what you can accomplish when you focus your energies on an established target.

3

Monitoring the Health of the Business

Keeping a business on course requires more than just good instincts. It's easy to get off track if you don't have a detailed plan. Although tracking business performance is essential, it takes time that many small practice owners and managers don't have. The fact is that most hearing health care professionals spend 99% of their time working *in* their businesses but little time working *on* their businesses. Some small business owners may believe they need to be around to get the business going, but once it is firmly established, it should pretty much run itself. However, if you want a good business, you will discover it won't just run itself. You may survive (and even thrive) in spite of yourself, but you won't have the business you could have if you don't watch your numbers.

One of the most important ways to determine the health of a business can be found in a profit and loss statement (P & L). This statement measures a company's sales and expenses during a specified period of time. The function of a P & L statement is to total all sources of revenue and subtract all expenses related to the revenue. It shows a company's financial progress during the time period being examined.

The P & L statement contains uniform categories of sales and expenses. The categories include, net sales, costs of goods sold, gross margin, administrative expense (or operating expense), salaries, and net profit. These are categories used to determine the health of a practice. Because it depicts a record of sales and expenses, the P & L statement will give a feel for the flows of cash in and out of a business.

If the goal is to make a profit, then you have to know how much revenue must be generated to make a profit. Consequently, it's essential to know the break-even point. The break-even point occurs when a business is neither making nor losing money. In other words—Total revenue = total expenses. Of course, the goal of any business is to generate a profit over and above the break-even point. Fixed costs exist regardless of how much revenue is generated. They include expenses like rent, employee wages, utilities, insurance, telephone, and Internet usage. Fixed expenses are bills that have to be paid every month. If you sell a product, the gross profit margin is the percentage of sales left after subtracting the cost of goods sold. There are many great resources and sample worksheets on the Internet to help determine the break-even point, and certainly an accountant can help (Table 3–1).

Key Performance Indicators (KPIs) are easy-to-implement tools that can simplify the process of monitoring the profitability of a business. A KPI is a measurable value that demonstrates how effectively a company is achieving key business objectives. KPIs are nothing more than a set of numbers used to evaluate the activity and performance of individuals working within your practice. KPIs, when properly utilized, are a proven approach to providing better patient outcomes, maintaining your best staff, generating more revenue, and being more profitable. Rather than making unsubstantiated judgements, a targeted set of KPIs allow you to make educated decisions about your practice. The most common KPIs usually include some variation of average selling price, units sold, units returned for credit, and opportunities to dispense products. Other KPIs can involve procedures in a practice, such as number of appointments scheduled per day and perhaps even revenue generated per patient visit.

The use of KPIs in the decision-making process and a focus on these numbers usually leads to better outcomes. However, success in a business doesn't just depend on numbers. Someone, usually an owner or manager, has to determine which KPIs to

Table 3–1. Example of a Budget

Gross revenue for a month	
Diagnostics and other service fees	9,000
Hearing aids 14 @ ASP $2200	30,800
Total Gross Revenue	39,800

Expenses for a month	
Audiologist Salary	7,000
One support staff	2,500
Hearing Aids COG 35%	10,780
Office Rent	2,500
Insurance	1,000
Loan Interest & Principal ($100,000)	4,800
Marketing	4,000
Misc. Expenses (utilities, supplies)	1,900
Total Expenses	34,480

Net revenue for the month	**5,320**

measure, and then uses those measurements to guide the daily operations of the business. KPIs, when measured and used properly, will provide a summary of crucial activity in the practice.

Many organizations use KPIs to evaluate their success at reaching targets. KPIs can provide a simple way to pare down an overwhelming amount of information into meaningful data, and will serve as a monthly report card of how well the business is performing.

As a business owner, I have become a numbers fanatic because I have found that looking at data is critical for making quick decisions, and essential for tracking the health of the business. It helps give me a feel for what's working and reveals areas that need to be improved. Unfortunately, some business owners do not track their numbers, and that is an easy way to get into financial trouble. I know everyone has a lot to do, but tracking certain key aspects of the business is absolutely necessary if you want to maintain a profitable business. I will offer a few suggestions of KPIs that are crucial to profitability of a practice.

If You Do One Thing and Only One Thing, Track Help Rate

Help Rate, or in sales terms it is called a Close Rate, is calculated by dividing the number of patients who purchase hearing aids by the total number of patients who were tested and received a recommendation for hearing aids. This is called a Close Rate in sales presentations. Increasing your Close or Help Rate by even a small percentage has the potential to dramatically impact the profitability of a practice.

Industry trends indicate that overall Help Rate in hearing health care practices is typically less than 50%. Although colleagues report that they convince 90% or more of patients who walk through their doors that they can benefit from hearing aids, to purchase them, the figures certainly don't support anything close to that number. I am sure you will agree that this is a very disturbing statistic. If you really want to improve profitability, start tracking your Help Rate and then commit to improving it. Just imagine the satisfaction you will feel at helping more patients hear better, not to mention the additional revenue you will generate. We all hear the same objections every day from our patients: "I don't think my hearing is bad enough;" "Hearing aids cost a lot of money;" "I want to think about it;" and "I need to talk with my spouse or my children." We should be prepared and not surprised by them. Learn how to handle these objections and your Help Rate will improve.

Professional convictions aside, imagine how revenue would grow in that average hearing health care practice if the professional focused on convincing more patients that need hearing aids to purchase them. According to Abram Bailey's industry survey of audiologists in 2018 (as reported on his hearingtracker.com website), the average practice dispensed 18 to 21 units per month. If Help Rates improved from the typical rate of less than 50% to 70%, revenue would increase by hundreds of thousands of dollars per year, based upon the average selling price per unit of $2372 (also reported by Bailey). The point is that helping more patients will positively impact your bottom line. Therefore, it seems obvious that focusing on improving your Help

Rate should be a priority. Additional information on overcoming objections is presented later in the guide.

There are several other KPIs that have the potential to add tremendous revenue to a practice.

Number of Hearing Aid Units Sold

Most private practices derive a large portion of their revenues from selling hearing aids. A simple barometer of the health of the business is whether the number of hearing aids sold is increasing or decreasing, compared to prior months or to the same point the prior year.

Cost of Goods Sold

The biggest expense is the cost of goods sold (COG) in the form of hearing aids. If your COG is more than 35%, it may be necessary to raise prices. If your prices are in line with the cost of doing business, then contact your suppliers and attempt to renegotiate prices. If a price reduction is not possible, try to negotiate free delivery, extended warranties, or extra receivers at no charge. Hearing aid sales by big box retailers are the fastest growing segment of the hearing aid market. An article written by Lee, Barrett, and Samuel in the December 2017 issue of *The Hearing Review* estimates Costco's U.S. market share to be around 11% of total sales, with the retailer's year-on-year unit growth increasing at an estimated 20% to 25% pace during the past 5 to 6 years, while the average audiology practice grew only 2% to 3%. At Costco, the largest wholesaler of hearing aids, devices often sell for less than audiologists pay for similar products, despite the fact that the aids are produced by the same manufacturing companies. So can audiologists win the price war? Economics would suggest that to compete on price alone, an average practice would need to see three times as many patients as they currently see to make up for the reduced margins created by the dramatically discounted prices offered by big box retailers, and on the internet. Where will those additional patients come from? How does a typical audiology practice compete against these giants? Perhaps the answer is not in waging a price war, but in creating a practice that focuses on the *Best in Hearing Health Care*.

Return for Credit

This statistic represents the number of hearing aids that were purchased by patients and returned for a refund. However, it may represent much more to the business, as it indicates the number of patients who were dissatisfied with the result provided by amplification, or with the way they were treated by personnel in the practice. When a patient returns an aid, dig in and investigate what the problem was so you can take steps to reduce returns in the future. I have found that setting a goal for "return for credit" has helped us significantly reduce the number of hearing aids returned to us. It's all in how the concept is presented to the patient. Telling patients that they have an Adjustment Period is much more effective than suggesting that they can "try" the aids and return them if they aren't satisfied.

Number of Patients Coming for an Evaluation Accompanied by a Third Party

It is difficult to help a person who comes to the appointment alone and denies that they have a problem. A third party helps reinforce the need for getting assistance for the hearing loss, and may eliminate possible objections to doing so. The person scheduling an appointment for a new patient or a previous patient coming for a reevaluation needs to actively solicit the third party by saying something like, "You will need to bring a person with a familiar voice to your appointment so Dr. Kasewurm can complete her testing." This is not an unsubstantiated request or just a sales tool. Hearing loss is about communication. A hearing device can certainly help a patient hear, but communication takes two people and can affect many other relationships. Asking for a third party to accompany a potential prospect is important for understanding the impact of hearing loss, and can also be good for business.

Percentage of Binaural Fittings

The last time I looked, a patient has two ears, and research indicates that patients with binaural hearing loss understand and hear better when wearing two hearing aids, so converting a monaural fitting into a binaural fitting can increase revenue and should also improve patient satisfaction.

Number of Calls Converted to Appointments

When a prospective patient calls your practice, the objective of the person who handles the call is to set an appointment. Every patient who calls and does not make an appointment represents potential lost revenue. You no longer have to wonder what a receptionist is saying. Call Source (http://www.callsource.com), or a similar call tracking service, can be an excellent resource that will actually record phone calls coming into your practice so you know how many incoming calls are being converted to appointments, and you can listen to what transpired to make certain calls are being answered properly. Tracking this KPI can also be as simple as having a tracking sheet at the front desk where the receptionist can record the number of calls versus the number of appointments scheduled.

Revenue Generated From Diagnostics

Most hearing health care practices generate revenue from diagnostic testing. A KPI based upon diagnostic revenue can be translated into the number of tests per day that need to be completed. This number should also take into account the reduction in reimbursement as a result of billing insurances.

Tracking KPIs can be a simple and effective way to determine the health of a business and whether it is growing or losing ground. Whatever KPIs you decide to measure, it is imperative that the data is accurate and easy to collect. This starts with having a computer-based office management system that can store and even analyze the data entered into the system. There are several computer-based office management systems (e.g., Sycle .net, Blueprint, Timms, CouncilEar) that are relatively inexpensive and affordable for all sized practices. Further, a computerized office management system typically offers reports that are simple and easy to run. KPIs can help a practice define and measure progress when the process includes setting goals. Consider the information in Table 3–2 as a place to start when setting goals for KPIs in your practice.

Table 3–2. Sample Key Performance Indicators (KPIs)

KPI
Total number of inbound calls converted to appointments Goal 98%
Total number of tests with a significant other or family member present Goal 65%
Binaural rate Goal 98%
Number of units sold/dispensed Depends on age of business and previous sales
Average selling price of units sold Goal $2250 per unit
Number of units returned Goal Less than 2%
Total net revenue Depends on practice

4

Innovative Marketing

At a recent social event, a physician approached me to discuss my marketing campaign. "How can you afford to market your business so much?" he asked. "I am a physician and I just don't have the funds to do that." At that moment, the muddy waters surrounding marketing became crystal clear and I realized that if you can't afford to market, you can't afford NOT to market.

Throughout the years, I have devised and executed countless marketing activities and spent more money than I care to remember, so I am always shocked when local residents tell me that despite operating my practice in the community for over thirty years, they have never heard of my practice. How could they not have noticed the hundreds of ads, direct mail pieces, radio spots, TV campaigns, educational seminars, internet marketing, community-sponsored events, and more, that we have done over the years?

On any given day, our current and prospective patients are bombarded with thousands of advertising messages in a wide array of mediums. So what's the best place to invest marketing dollars? I am not really sure, but what I am convinced of is that attracting new patients is getting more and more complicated and expensive, and if your marketing efforts aren't producing results, then it's important to pull the plug, and try something new. Of course, you won't know how expensive it is to attract a new patient if you aren't tracking and measuring the results of each campaign you run.

27

Although I don't I have a crystal ball, I will let you in on what we have discovered in the marketing efforts at my practice. Our typical external monthly marketing campaign combines direct mail, print, radio, television, social media, and other digital marketing. While response to direct mail has definitely decreased in recent years, it still proves effective as part of the marketing mix for my practice. My industry contacts tell me that the average cost for every call that results from a marketing campaign should be no more than $320. When ours climbed much higher than that, we reevaluated and discovered that our print advertising was no longer working and prospective patients were no longer calling as a result of the large display ads in the newspaper. Although we were uncertain whether it was the medium or the message, we pulled the newspaper ads and moved those dollars into social media ads on a *local celebrity's* website. This individual happens to be a local radio personality whom we fit with hearing aids, and he does "ad libs" on his show that talk about my practice and the benefits of better hearing. Advertising on his website seemed a natural companion to the radio messages. Although we stopped the display ads, we have experienced some success with "sticky note" ads in our local newspaper and they were less expensive than display ads. Television spots still seem to be reaching our demographic if they are run at the right times. Previous campaigns consisted of hundreds of monthly ads run through the day and night. However, what's the point of running an ad at 2 AM or 10 PM if a patient can't pick up the phone to make an appointment when he or she hears the ad? We continue to see results from our television spots, but only when they are run during the hours the office is open in order that patients can call immediately to schedule an appointment. Potential patients may not remember or may they have reconsidered if they have to wait until the office is open.

Our marketing campaigns continue to include a direct mail component, but the response is diminishing. The days of gleaning a .01% or even half of .01% response are over, but a letter with a coupon at the bottom continues to draw a reasonable and cost-effective response from prospects at this time in my practice.

Today, more than ever, consumers are bombarded with marketing messages, so it should not be surprising when a marketing piece goes unnoticed. If your marketing budget is limited, and most are, and you want to use your dollars effectively, you will need to carefully plan a campaign to reach your target audience. This will not be an easy task. It's a painstaking process that requires time, energy, and constant reevaluation. The general rule of thumb is if you want to grow, you have to market. Although I measure and monitor the outcomes of every marketing effort, I have yet to find one thing that consistently brings new patients through the door. So, how does one know how much to spend and where to spend it when it comes to marketing? There's no crystal ball that provides a simple answer to that question. However, I have read that an established practice should invest 5 to 8% of gross revenue in a marketing budget. New practices may have to invest more to get started.

Marketing Is More than Advertising

Marketing is the process that involves everything you do to promote your business or organization. A simple way to distinguish between marketing and advertising is to think of marketing as a pie and inside that pie you have slices of advertising, market research, media planning, public relations, product pricing, distribution, customer support, sales strategy, and community involvement. Although advertising is only a small piece of the pie, it's usually the ingredient that costs the most.

The essence of marketing is to understand patients' needs and to develop a plan that caters to those needs. Although it is difficult to find ways to reach a target market, perhaps we should stop searching for instant gratification and start hunting for a purple cow. What in the world is a purple cow, you may ask? It's finding *new* and *unique* ways to reach your ideal patient. Many of us are so in need of a quick fix and instant gratification that we use the same old ads to get patients in our doors for a sale or an open house. Patients sometimes come into my office with bags of such ads all promoting the same things, such as discounted prices, or looking for "Wanted: twenty people to try something new." We have all seen and heard it before. It's time to think of something *new* and *exciting* that will make a prospect want to act *now* to take that first step of making an appointment for a hearing evaluation. Although I have completed many, many marketing activities in thirty years, I am not an expert on the best ways to reach your target audience. That is why I recommend hiring a marketing consultant or talking with your manufacturing partners to learn the most effective ways to reach your target market.

It's been my experience that many hearing health care providers utilize Infusion Marketing. When we need an instant infusion of patients, we run an ad offering free screenings or special discounts for a short period of time. Although this "Come now and get it while it's hot" promotion may work for the moment, it's doesn't solve the long-term problem of consistently promoting the image of the business. There's no quick fix when it comes to successful marketing.

The first step in a marketing effort is to develop a strategy that will form a solid foundation for everything you do to promote your business or organization. Implementing promotional activities such as print ads, direct mail, pay-per-click campaigns, educational seminars, or even networking without a marketing strategy is like buying curtains for a house you are building before you have an architectural plan. How would you know how many curtains to buy or what size they need to be? Take some time to develop a plan that will serve as a guide for all of your marketing efforts throughout the year. The plan should be specific to the types of activities conducted, how often they will be executed, and the expected outcomes.

Once a marketing strategy has been developed, the next step is to develop a budget. When you establish a budget, you are making a commitment to spend a set amount of money to promote your business or organization. How much should you spend? That depends on how much you want to gain. As mentoned earlier, marketing experts suggest that 5% to 8% of gross revenues should be allocated for marketing. The more you spend, the more you have to gain. However, this is true only if the marketing efforts yield positive results. Although not every effort may be equally successful, as long as the effort generates more revenue than you spend, it can be considered a successful marketing effort.

Everyone or anybody might be potential patients. However, you probably don't have the time or money to market to everyone or anybody. Many business owners fall into the trap of believing that their products or services are "for everyone"—that is, anyone would be interested in or need the products. Even though people with hearing loss represent a broad and diverse market, you need to identify who your ideal patient is. After you've identified your primary market, your advertising should match that focus. Identify specific groups that make sense to spend your time and money promoting your business or organization to, and then plan a strategy to go out and get them!

Once you have developed a strategy and a plan, it's time to determine the focus of the message. A good marketing strategy should have a common theme that permeates every marketing activity, regardless of the medium. What is it that established and potential patients are really seeking? You may be offering balance testing, hearing assessments, and many types of amplification, but potential patients are also purchasing better relationships, improved communication, increased productivity, enhanced self-esteem, and a less stressful life. All marketing efforts should promote the benefits of better hearing. It's not about who YOU are, but rather about who the PATIENT wants to become when he or she is able to hear better.

Too often, hearing health care professionals only market when they need business. Marketing involves more than placing an ad or setting up and editing a website. Ongoing, consistent, and creative efforts must be made to promote a business. Some experts suggest that being consistent has a greater impact than the specific message that is offered. This, in part, is the reason for the success of chains. Whether you're going to Little Rock, Arkansas, or New York City, if you reserve a room at a Courtyard Marriott, you know exactly what you're going to get, just as your marketing campaign should explain to patients what they are going to get when they visit your practice.

Finally, it's crucial that you measure and monitor every marketing activity so you know what works in your particular setting. If the message isn't reaching your target market, review your plan and change the message. You certainly don't want to invest hard-earned dollars in a campaign that isn't reaching your audience. Before developing a brochure, running an ad, executing a direct mail campaign, implementing a pay-per-click activity, or presenting an educational seminar, ask yourself if you have outlined a clear, consistent marketing strategy. If the answer is, "no," take the time to outline a plan that will potentially set a new course for your business or organization.

Every marketing piece has to have a strong call to action. You have to give someone a reason to pick up that phone *today* and call for an appointment. After all, most new patients wait six to eight years after they notice some difficulties hearing to make an appointment, so what's the reason to finally take action and call *now*? What do you have that the big box stores don't have? Try to highlight what makes your company unique in your marketing materials. Make your unique brand of hearing health care very clear to your prospects by emphasizing quality, experience, and service.

It's All About the Buzz

As a confirmed sugar freak, I am on a continual pursuit for the ultimate confectionary. Following a great dinner in New York City, I found myself craving a sweet treat. When I shared my urge with a friend, she assured me that she knew of the perfect spot to indulge my craving. We rushed to the closest subway station and rode 82 blocks before reaching our destination. I know New Yorkers are late-nighters, but I had to wonder how good this place must be to travel so far at 11 o'clock at night.

When we arrived at the infamous Magnolia Bakery, it was obvious by the throngs of people lined up around the building that this must be a very special place if people were willing to wait in line and pay an outrageous price for a cupcake at this time of night. There was even a bouncer to control the crowd. As I perused the lively group, I had to wonder, how can I create this kind of excitement about my business? I can't imagine that an average patient with an appointment at a hearing health care office would even consider standing in line to have her or his hearing tested. In fact, it is not unusual to have to bribe patients with some type of special offer to get them to walk through our doors. So how can we generate the same type of excitement about better hearing that Magnolia Bakery has created for their cupcakes?

Marketing guru, Seth Godin, suggests that it takes a remarkable or even bizarre idea to get a consumer's attention. Tired of seeing the same old messages about price and cosmetics? Chances are, so is everyone else. Marketing pieces can get tired and worn-out looking if used too often. If you have been using the same message for an extended period of time, create something new. Instead of promoting products, promote the benefits of better hearing. Ask patients to do testimonials about how much they love hearing better and then use them in your marketing materials. Try a newspaper insert instead of a printed ad. Instead of sending generic direct mail pieces, send something that your audience will remember, such as a package of M&M's with a note that says, "What do our hearing aids and this candy have in common? Call our office today to find out." It's color, in case you are wondering.

Try offering a new service or product. Millions of consumers are walking around with something in their ears these days. Expand your target market by offering and promoting something that appeals to a larger audience, such as custom Bluetooth earpieces for cellular phones, or OTCs that serve as hearing enhancers and an entry into the market.

Insurance companies are reducing reimbursements and encouraging subscribers to change to Internet Third Party Providers (TPAs). In an effort to make up for business lost to these entities, we have developed relationships with local companies, and have become preferred providers for their employees. Many of these companies allow us to present to their employees, and we place advertorials in their employee newsletters. We have also found success becoming preferred providers for local companies that offer hearing health benefits to their employees. I have included promotional pieces that we have developed for these companies (Figure 4–1).

Patient Referral Program

Word-of-mouth marketing can be the biggest influence on people to buy, or not to buy, products and services. Satisfied patients are usually the best advocates for a business, but many business owners often fail to ask them to spread the word. Our Patient Referral Program continues to provide a large percentage of our new patients. A referral from a family member or friend is still viewed by patients as the most trusted source when making a major buying decision, such as whether to purchase hearing aids.

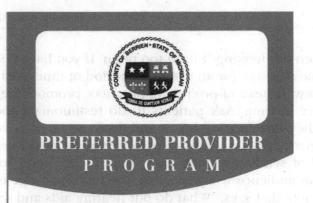

PREFERRED PROVIDER
P R O G R A M

At **Dr. Kasewurm's Professional Hearing Services**, we believe the quality of your hearing directly affects the quality of your life. That's why we're proud to partner with the **County of Berrien** to offer you our free **Preferred Provider Program**.

This valuable and convenient program was designed to help you find the best solution for your hearing needs and lifestyle – at the best value.

It gives you and your family access to free hearing screenings, significant discounts on hearing aids, and more.

Our staff is dedicated to providing you with the highest quality hearing healthcare. We take pride in offering services and solutions specifically designed around your individualized needs.

Our **Preferred Provider Program** is proof of our commitment to helping you and your loved ones hear your best.

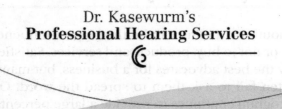

Dr. Kasewurm's
Professional Hearing Services

Figure 4–1. Example of a Preferred Provider promotional card.

34

In my practice, we find that patients referred by other patients are more likely to purchase at the time of their first visit AND are willing to invest more for better hearing.

Many of my friends and colleagues tell me they have referral programs, but I have found that most programs aren't specific enough. To be successful, the program has to be very specific and intentional. It's not enough to simply tell your staff to "ask for referrals." I recently ran into a friend I hadn't seen in some time and we both agreed that we needed to make a date to get together, but we never set up something specific. The odds of reconnecting with that old friend are slim.

Referrals from patients don't happen automatically. You have to make them happen and that means having specific goals that you regularly monitor and push to achieve. I don't believe in just sitting by and waiting for the phone to ring. I know what I want for the practice, and I set goals and motivate the entire staff to help make success happen. Our program includes having each team member put five referral cards in his pocket each morning with an expiration date of no more than one month out, and the goal is to distribute those five cards each day.

A paragraph on our Patient Referral Program is included in each of our newsletters, and includes a testimonial by a patient who came to our office because of the gentle nudging of another patient. The testimonials don't have to be lengthy to be effective —about 250 words is plenty. To take this a step further, we video-tape these joyful musings and put them on our website. Infusing new patients into a practice through a patient referral program can be an effective and efficient way to increase revenue. I have materials to help you start a Patient Referral Program that I am happy to share if you write to me at http://www.DrGyl.com

If you don't have a formal patient referral program, start one. Print cards with your name, address, and phone number and ask patients to hand them out to their friends and family. It's been my experience that the cards are most effective if they have an expiration date no longer than 30 days in the future. The best time to hand out referral cards is when a patient expresses their satisfaction with the products or services you have provided. Patients are usually happy to tell their friends and relatives about you, but it is unlikely to happen unless it is an *intentional* effort. Set a goal to hand out a specific number of cards every day and set goals for your staff to do the same. A successful patient referral program can provide a revenue boost for a practice. When a patient who has been referred comes in for an appointment, send a personal note to the patient who referred the new person and tell them how much it means to you and the business. You may want to have exclusive events for members of your referral club. We have had great success with our Patient Referral Program, which now accounts for 70% of new business for the practice.

Patient Events

Special events in a practice can attract attention and a new audience. Plan an event, like a golf tournament, and invite patients and prospects to participate, or purchase tickets to a show or concert and ask your patients to invite their friends. We once held a Wild Wednesday program on the first Wednesday of every month when we served refreshments and offered demonstrations of the latest hearing technology, and encouraged patients to invite their friends to attend. Consider an Open House in which you don't promote a product, but you serve refreshments instead and offer advice about hearing loss in a very non-threatening environment? We have hosted spaghetti dinners that served as fundraisers for charitable organizations. Patients like to feel special and holding events for "patients only" can promote positive emotions towards you and your business.

Staying in Touch With Patients

A newsletter is another wonderful way to distribute information to your existing patient base, and an excellent way to reach out to prospective patients and other professionals regarding the services and products you provide. A newsletter can be a beneficial and cost-effective investment for your business or organization. Whether you're using a newsletter to boost sales and referrals, or to educate readers, you would attempt to generate enough revenue to offset the costs of publishing and distributing the newsletter. In many cases, it will be more cost effective to enlist the services of an outside vendor to create and publish an electronic newsletter. A newsletter should generate a return on investment that is worth the cost and time to produce the newsletter and can serve as one of the four necessary communications that you should have with your patients every year.

A newsletter can focus the reader on useful or new information, but the goal is to generate results. Articles should be chosen for their ability to attract interest in new products or services, or on providing answers to frequently asked questions. A newsletter is also a way to advertise any specials, promotions, or seminars that you may be offering in the near future. Newsletters that fill pages with generic "filler" items, such as recipes and famous quotations may be bulky, but not effective. Small newsletters, even as little as a page or two, can be just as effective in relaying important and interesting information to your readers. Topics can include information on the latest research, updates on new technology, attendance at conventions or educational programs, new hours, or special celebrations of staff members.

Newsletters can be created monthly, quarterly, or annually. However, some hearing health care professionals find it helpful to send shorter, monthly newsletters to keep in touch with their patients. The newsletter can be created using simple software such as Microsoft Publisher®.

In addition to creating the newsletter, customizing the message for different categories of your patient database (i.e., current patients, prospects, tested but not sold, etc.) is essential. For instance, you may not want to send a newsletter that contains information on a new technology to patients who purchased new aids within the past few months. Or you may want to produce a newsletter for your pediatric patients. The purpose of any patient communication is to keep your patients connected to you and your organization and to let them know that you are keeping abreast of the latest technological and clinical developments. If you don't tell your patients and prospects about the latest advancements for hearing loss, you can bet your competitors will. People are living longer and developing hearing loss at younger ages, so the lifetime value of every patient is increasing, so it's important to stay in touch.

Patient retention has become critical to the success of a practice. What are you doing to ensure patients stay with you? Scheduling regular patient visits is a good way to retain patients and to ensure they get the care they need. I might suggest annual hearing tests and cleanings every six months for hearing aids. I have found great success in including batteries in the price of a "better hearing package," which keeps patients returning to us for their *free* batteries. The "power of free" can be incredibly attractive to people and can influence the choice for a hearing health care provider. Stay in touch with your patients and let them know you appreciate them. Attempt to contact them four times a year: 6-month cleaning, annual evaluations, and perhaps a newsletter and a birthday card.

> **Price is what you Pay, but Value is What you Get.**

Digital Marketing

Digital marketing has become increasingly more important and is only going to become more of a factor in years to come. We have had great success attracting new patients with Facebook ads.

Although it has become increasingly popular to advertise on social media, I can't help but notice that there are a much greater number of ads. Facebook advertising is certainly easy and inexpensive but it still requires constant tracking to make sure you are getting a good return on the investment. A recent ad that cost my business $1000 over a month's time produced 133 leads. However, what we have discovered is that it takes up to five contacts to reach a lead, and it's important to follow up on the lead as soon after it is posted as possible; only 30% of the leads actually make appointments, and then only half of the appointments actually show up. I have confirmed these stats with other practice owners and it seems to be consistent.

Don't forget to include e-mail marketing, social media, and your website to let prospects and patients know about your upcoming events. Make sure any offers have clear calls to action.

When someone lands on your website, you have mere seconds to grab his or her attention. Don't make visitors have to search for what they want—put it directly in front of them. Structure your e-mail autoresponder, and there are many programs available on the internet such as Constant Contact or Mail Chimp, sequences to "touch" your leads more frequently during the holiday season, and don't be afraid to send more direct-promotional offers.

Make sure your website is mobile friendly. According to entrepreneur.com, 28.9% of all internet traffic in 2017 came from mobile devices. First, run your website pages through Google's mobile-friendly test to make sure the search engine deems your pages mobile friendly. Although this gives a good indication, you need to take it a step further. Ask employees, friends, and family to run through your website on their mobile devices and provide you with honest feedback.

Common Marketing Mistakes

With so many mediums available, marketing continues to be a conundrum. What will work? What won't work and how much will I have spent to find out? Marketing is important because you need it to grow a business, but it can be a huge endeavor and one that's difficult to fit into a schedule when you are also seeing patients and running the business.

It isn't financially prudent to try to attract *everyone* and *anyone* into your business. Many businesses know their products and services up and down but have only a vague idea of who might actually want or need them. It's important to know who your ideal patient is and go after that demographic. In my practice, we target people over the age of 60 years with a minimum household income of $40,000. You will also need to know the radius you want to target and the number of total marketing pieces that you want and can afford to send.

Every marketing piece should give the reader a reason to act NOW! Even when marketers DO understand their target audience, they often have an extraordinarily difficult time formulating a value proposition that gives readers a reason to pick up the phone and call today. For example:

Good: "Call us today to be the first to experience this new technology. This offer is only valid through . . . " It doesn't really matter what the offer is—a specialist coming to town on a specific date or a discount for a short time period.

Not So Good: "Give us a call for a free sample." This example doesn't create the urgency to call NOW. I recently ran across an old marketing piece and there was no call to action and the result was a lot of money spent with no response.

I cannot stress enough the importance of tracking the results of every campaign. You certainly don't want to throw money away on campaigns that fail to get new patients to walk through your doors. I can hear people out there saying, "Come on Dr. Gyl. How can we possibly do one more thing?" No worries as YOU don't have to be the person tracking the results. Your reception-ist can track where every new patient comes from, or you may want to consider using a call-tracking service. Most electronic software will provide sales generated by referral source as long as the source is entered into the software.

There is no one-stop shopping when it comes to marketing. You have to try multiple mediums to see what works, and when you find something that works, I suggest that you keep doing it until it doesn't work anymore. I have spoken with many col-leagues that ask, "Can you send me your marketing pieces that are working?" There is no simple answer. What works in my area may not work in another market.

5

Creating an Experience to Remember

In today's world, the patient experience is everything! Some years ago, I recall reading that "the patient experience is fast becoming the next competitive battleground in healthcare." In today's competitive marketplace, an organization's brand is built—or broken—on the patient experience. In fact, according to the *Customers 2020* study by Walker, a customer intelligence consulting firm in the United States, by 2020 the customer experience will overtake price and product as the key brand differentiator.

My recent birthday brought to mind the need for my yearly physical. Although I dreaded the annual exam, I was hopeful the visit to a new, young female doctor might be better than my previous experiences.

The office was one of many in a new, large medical facility, but the lack of signage failed to point a clear route to my physician's office. When I finally located the office, the receptionist barely glanced my way, handed me a clipboard and instructed me to "take a seat and fill this out." Rather surprising as I had already completed mounds of paperwork before the visit. When I didn't see an obvious coat rack, I asked where I could hang my wet coat. "I guess you'll have to hold it," snapped the young woman as she gazed down at a fitness magazine.

The clock ticked by as my appointment time came and went with no explanation from anyone. At last, the nurse arrived and announced to everyone in the waiting room, "*Gill* Kasewurm, you can come back and get on the scale now." "My name is *Jill*," I said sheepishly. "Sorry, *Gill*," she snapped. "Follow me."

For those of you old enough to have seen *One Flew Over the Cuckoo's Nest*, "Nurse Ratchet" led me to a stark white room and instructed me to, "Put this on with the V in front." Because both sides of the very small garment had what appeared to be a V, I looked up to ask for clarification only to see the door close in my face. This experience was going from bad to worse and I hadn't even seen the stirrups yet. There was no way I was going to recommend this physician to anyone and I hadn't even met her yet! This gave me reason to wonder what type of experience my patients encounter when they visit my practice.

Unless we take steps to manage how patients are treated in our offices, mistakes like these are sure to happen. Considering that the goal is to keep patients for a lifetime, we must be intentional in ensuring the patient experience is one that is positive and makes patients want to return and tell others about the wonderful encounter.

Research indicates that consumers are willing to pay more for an extraordinary experience. What do Starbucks, Disneyland and Apple Computer have in common? The answer is experience, and I am not referring to how long they have been in business. The following are some suggestions on how you can improve the experience for your patients.

Ensure a Good First Impression

I recently had the privilege of visiting the Chianti region of Italy, where our travels included a visit to several wineries. Although the countryside was beautiful and the wine was great, I found myself a bit bored after the second winery. A winery is a winery, right? That's what I thought until our group reached Casa Emma.

As we approached the remote vineyard, a young Italian man stood in the driveway gleefully waving his arms to welcome us.

As he led us on our tour, he explained that Casa Emma was no ordinary winery. His unbridled enthusiasm was so captivating that I found myself riveted on his every word. By the end of the tour, I was convinced that this little-known winery was indeed the best in Italy. I left with a happy heart (it wasn't just the wine) wondering how my staff and I could make patients feel as good about my practice as this fellow made me feel about Casa Emma.

First impressions are lasting ones and the first impression of you and your practice is often given by the person managing the front desk and answering the phone. Therefore, it's crucial that this employee is enthusiastic and well trained to handle the job. Accomplishing this will require supervision and ongoing training. If you want to ensure that your current and potential patients are made to feel welcomed and appreciated every time they call or visit your office, it's crucial that the staff member at the front desk is a "people person."

Hire Friendly People

You can train a person to do a job but you can't train a person to be genuinely nice. An employee who handles the front desk may be highly qualified, but if he or she is incapable of engaging patients in light conversation, he or she may be perceived as unfriendly or indifferent. A receptionist must understand how valuable she or he is to the organization and should recognize the important role she or he holds in establishing and maintaining relationships with patients.

Training sessions should be held regularly on how to greet patients, as well as on how to be attentive to their individual needs. A good receptionist must have the ability to create a sense of warmth and comfort for patients, not unlike the feeling you would want to give good friends when they enter your home. Something as simple as a smile can go a long way to make a person feel welcomed and appreciated.

The employee who greets patients and answers your phone should be trained to correctly answer patients' most common questions and concerns. A potential patient may have fears about having a hearing evaluation and will resist making an appointment until he is reassured that it is simple and painless.

Potential patients often call to inquire about the cost of hearing aids and the answer can determine whether or not they make an appointment. Keep in mind, if a person is calling in response to an advertisement, you have considerable dollars already invested in the caller and that investment will be lost if no appointment is scheduled. I would recommend composing a script for front desk personnel so they have the available tools to answer the most commonly asked questions. It's a good idea to actually practice those questions and answers with your front office personnel to ensure that they feel comfortable and confident with those discussions. I have included some sample scripts at the end of this guide.

Front office personnel should be familiar with the services you provide in your practice. Take some time to run a complete test battery on your receptionist. Callers often inquire about what they can expect to encounter during their appointment and front desk personnel should be able to outline what the potential patient may experience while in your office.

Potential patients don't have to look far to see an advertisement for hearing aids, and they may call to inquire about specific technologies before making an appointment. The responses to these technology questions can lead to unrealistic expectations if they are not answered appropriately. When a new product is released, include front desk personnel in the training and try to incite in them the same enthusiasm that you have for the new technology.

As the first point of contact for patients, the person handling your front desk and answering your phone is a direct reflection of your practice as a whole. Take some specific steps to make sure he or she shares your enthusiasm for better hearing with every person who contacts or visits the practice. Lost appointments represent lost revenue, so spending time to train and orient front desk personnel in the services you offer is well worth it.

A good patient experience just doesn't happen. You have to take deliberate and intentional steps to ensure that every patient experience is a positive one. Excessive wait times are not conducive to a positive patient experience. When a patient does have to wait, make sure she or he is informed of the anticipated wait time and give them the option of rescheduling when the wait time becomes excessive. Patients will usually exercise patience when they see someone busily helping another patient, but they may not be so understanding when they see an empty waiting room and feel ignored. I contend that patients don't mind waiting for a professional they like and trust but they do mind the unexpected. So, if you are forced to make a patient wait, let them know the reason and give them an idea of the length of the wait. When the wait gets excessive, give patients the opportunity to come back or reschedule at a time that is convenient for them, not you. If there is a scheduling error, admit you made a mistake, ask the patient when they would like to return, and then make certain you are on time for their next appointment.

Another step towards a positive patient experience is to avoid making patients complete piles of redundant paperwork. Take the opportunity to ask questions during the initial interview and ask for updates verbally when patients return for reevaluations. Consider sending intake forms and practice brochures to patients before their first visit and include directions to your office. You may also want to make the intake forms accessible on your website so patients can complete and send them before their appointment. If there isn't adequate time to send paperwork prior to the appointment, you could have an iPad for patients to input their information into your system, or the receptionist could verbally ask for the information to avoid making the patient complete cumbersome paperwork.

Your waiting room and treatment rooms should look warm and inviting, with comfortable and clean furniture. Although you may not have the funds or the authority to redecorate, a coat of fresh paint, especially in a warm color, can brighten an office. Offer creature comforts like coffee, water, and fresh cookies or other refreshments. Some of our patients arrive 30 minutes early just to relax and enjoy our freshly baked cookies. I have definitely gone to the extreme in creating a unique patient experience in my practice, but it has paid off by attracting word-of-mouth marketing because patients enjoy the atmosphere and tell others about it.

Listen and stay in good communication while the patient is in your office and after she or he leaves. It is beneficial to make note of personal details or a special interest of a patient that you can refer to later. Patients trust professionals who look them in the eye when discussing hearing test results and making recommendations. Nothing builds good will as much as looking a patient in the eye, shaking hands, and extending a sincere "thank you" for choosing you as their hearing health care provider. Patients have many choices and it's important to let patients know they are appreciated.

Moving from providing services to providing experiences may be just what separates you from your competition. In the age of the experience economy, patients themselves become the product. Make certain that the experiences you provide are ones that not only transform your patients' hearing, but also their lives.

Hearing health care professionals have LOTS of hurdles to overcome these days. It should be fun and easy to focus on your patient's experience, and to make it one to remember (Figures 5–1 through 5–5).

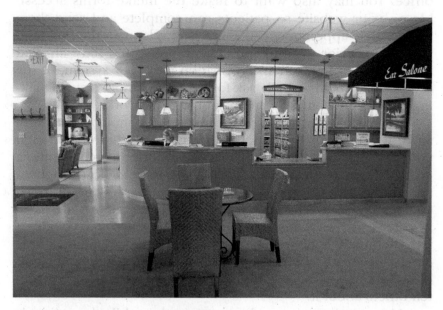

Figure 5–1. Front desk area at PHS.

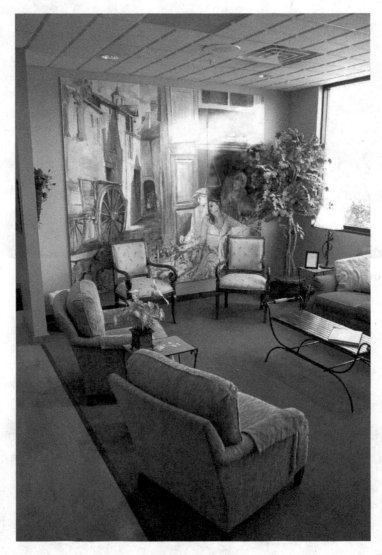

Figure 5–2. New patient gathering area at PHS.

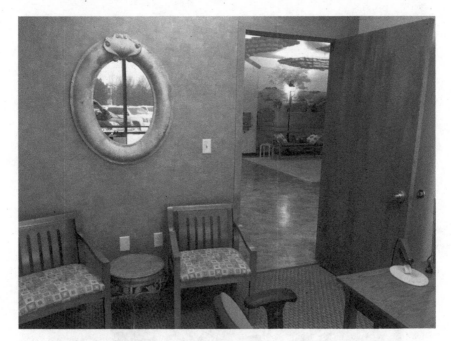

Figure 5–3. Treatment room décor at PHS.

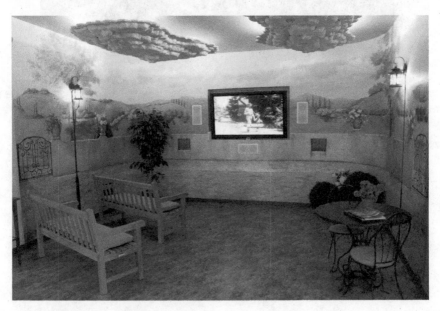

Figure 5–4. "Park" where we do presentations at PHS.

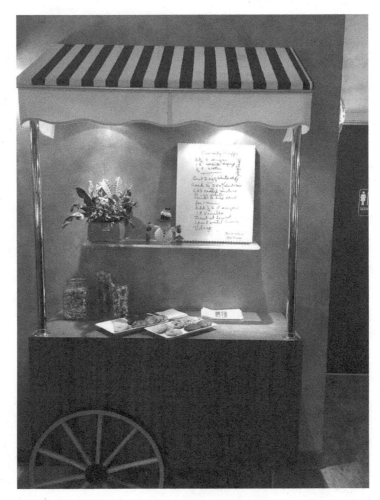

Figure 5–5. Cookies baked fresh daily at PHS.

6

Highlighting Patient Retention

While reviewing a spreadsheet that detailed patients' most recent visits to my office, I was dismayed to discover how many patients with whom we had lost touch. Considering the lifetime value of a patient, this represents a significant loss of potential revenue. Patient retention is vital to the success of any business and hearing health care is certainly no exception. In an industry that has had minimal growth in the past few years, just imagine what an increase in patient retention can mean to the profitability of a hearing health care business. So, how can we improve patient retention?

One way of growing a business is to increase sales to current patients, and marketing to current patients should be a part of every marketing plan. Are there additional products or services you can offer patients? An extended service program has the potential to not only add to your bottom line, but also to keep patients connected to you and your practice. I have seen colleagues offer several levels of service plans and to rename their contract as a Hearing Enhancement Plan that includes service plans, as well as technology, instead of simply including hearing devices.

The more patients know about you and your accomplishments, the more they will see you as a professional they can trust. Let patients know when you or a member of your staff completes an educational course. As a rule of thumb, try to communicate with your patients at least four times a year. Whether it is an e-mail newsletter, monthly flier, a reminder card for an annual hearing evaluation, or a holiday greeting card, reach out to your patients and let them know you care and want them to come back. Make sure to include notifications about new technology as well. If you aren't telling your patients about new technology, you can bet everyone else is!

When patients aren't happy with your business they usually won't complain to you. Instead, they'll probably complain to just about everyone else they know and take their business to your competition next time. Take steps to ensure patients are satisfied by making follow-up calls or mailing satisfaction questionnaires after the patient has visited your office, and then respond to any and all concerns that a patient makes on their survey (Figure 6–1).

Building patient loyalty will be a lot easier if you have a loyal workforce. It is especially important to retain employees who interact with patients on a regular basis. I've been fortunate to have the same great people in customer service for years, and the compliments from patients make it clear that they appreciate seeing the same familiar faces in our service department.

Maintaining an Exceptional Staff

I am often asked what the key is to operating a successful practice. Certainly, being a top notch professional is first, but running a close second is having an employee who is friendly, efficient, and capable of performing a multitude of duties in the practice. Most practitioners employ at least one person in addition to themselves. In a busy practice, this employee becomes a key component of the success of the practice. Duties may include everything from scheduling, to billing, to making minor hearing aid repairs, and even calming patients' nerves before their hearing evaluations. The key employee could also be involved in areas that lead to increased patient satisfaction by being aware of repair histories and recurring problems that a patient may be having.

We Want to Hear From You!

(Name),

Our mission is to provide you with the absolute best service. We are very interested in your experience with your hearing aid(s) as an evaluation of our performance. Please take a moment to fill out this short survey and return to us one week from today.

Thank you in advance and we look forward to hearing from you soon.

Sincerely,

Please rate the following Hearing Aid Features & Service Factors	Satisfied	Neutral	Dissatisfied
Overall fit/comfort			
Whistling/feedback/buzzing			
Understanding television			
The sound of your voice			
Ability to hear soft sounds			
Comfort with loud sounds			
Hearing in noisy situations			
Using the telephone			
Professionalism of provider			
Explanation on use and care of aid(s)			
Explanation of what to expect from aid(s)			
Convenience of our office hours			
How likely is it that you would recommend Professional Hearing Services to a friend?			

What services could we offer to assist you on your journey to better hearing?

_____

_____

Figure 6–1. Patient satisfaction survey.

Although the duties may vary by practice setting, there is no doubt that this employee is a *key* component of a successful practice, and if utilized properly, can lead the practice to another level of success. This *key* person may hold the title of receptionist, but regardless of the title, the role remains the same: to develop good patient relationships, generate leads from current patients, and ensure efficient and effective office procedures. Having a key employee should allow an owner or manager to spend more time doing what he or she does best, which is providing exceptional patient care and generating sufficient revenue to make the practice profitable.

One very important task for a key employee is to squeeze every productive moment out of the schedule. Let the employee know your expectations for scheduling and help them understand the need to confirm appointments at least 24 hours in advance, preferably 48 hours, and then to make every effort to fill last-minute cancellations. Every open appointment time is a potential loss of revenue. An employee who can skillfully juggle the busy schedule of a productive office is a valuable asset. However, some employees fail to hustle to fill vacancies because they don't see it as a priority and actually may think you really enjoy the free time. Although most practice owners and managers can easily fill open time to work on various aspects of the business, too many open appointments can ultimately lead to the death of a practice. A skilled scheduler who is informed can help avoid unnecessary last-minute drop-ins, without denying legitimate appointments.

The way your phone is answered may not be something you give a lot of thought or attention to, but it can have a tremendous impact on a patient's opinion of a practice. Ever been caught in the seemingly endless loop of an automated system? Press 1 for this and 2 for this and 12 for . . . . Imagine using such a system when you have difficulty hearing! A telephone call is often the first real impression a potential patient has of you and your organization. Sure, they might be familiar with your name, have driven by your office, or visited your website, but a phone call is typically the first real interaction a potential patient has with his hearing health care professional. Whether this experience is warm, positive, and memorable is highly dependent upon the individual who answers the phone in the practice. The right person can make all the difference in the world, whereas the wrong person can drive potential patients away forever. Good and repeatable telephone etiquette isn't automatic but rather something you should discuss and even practice with a key employee.

A key employee can assist with marketing, handling your personal schedule, calling manufacturers to order supplies, checking on orders, staying in touch with patients, and many other functions that will allow you to spend more quality time with your patients. If you are wondering what an average wage is for a key employee, check the latest Occupational Outlook Handbook http://www.bls.gov/ooh/ to learn what a typical pay scale is for your particular state. Talented key employees can more than pay for themselves through their contribution to the growth and success of a practice. The key employee can also serve as a patient recall specialist by going through the records and recalling patients who haven't been in for a reevaluation, and may be candidates for new hearing technology. Compensation may include bonuses for getting patients you have lost touch with back into the practice. A key employee truly represents the key components of a practice's success and should be well compensated if her or his performance is benefiting and enhancing the practice or organization.

Employees should be building relationships with patients that keep them coming back to the practice. Make sure to appreciate good employees and reward them for being loyal to you and your organization. In addition, empower employees to make decisions that benefit patients and encourage them to solve problems or complaints as quickly as possible. Excuses such as, "That's the boss's policy," or "Sorry, I am not allowed to do that" may turn a patient away permanently.

According to industry statistics and personnel experience, as few as 3% of tested-not-sold (TNS) prospects return to the same practice when they decide to purchase hearing aids. As a result, it's important to follow up with TNS prospects immediately following the initial contact with another contact 10 to 14 days later. You can then stay in touch every few months for the first year and then annually. Try to create a memorable message that will cause the patient to reconsider you and your practice for their hearing services. For instance, I read that someone sent a lottery ticket with a letter stating, "Take a chance on better hearing." The tactic isn't as important as the effort and letting the patient know that you want to be the one to help them with their hearing loss. The TNS prospects have the greatest potential for adding value to a business, but it's been my experience that the initial contact is the best opportunity to help the patient, and that opportunity diminishes over time.

Most hearing health care practices are small businesses with only a few employees. Just as every member of an athletic team plays a valuable role, the same is true of the players in a hearing health care office. If the professional is a wonderful clinician, but the receptionist insults patients, the team doesn't work. So, how can you create a team effort?

I was browsing through some old files the other day and I stumbled upon the exit interview of a former employee. When asked what would have improved her employment, she responded, "A few words of praise go a long way." After some soul searching, I had to wonder, "In my efforts to be in charge, have I been a team breaker, instead of a team maker?" Because I wasn't blessed with natural athletic abilities, I didn't gather my team building strategies from athletic coaches. However, as the boss in my business, I now find myself in the position of having to be a team leader. You have to be a secure person to be a leader. Leave your insecurities at home and grab all the strength you can muster to motivate your coworkers and colleagues to do their best. Give every member of the team the opportunity and freedom to grow and thrive in their work environments. You can't begin to build a strong and successful team without well-written job descriptions. Sometimes I expect my employees to simply know what I want done, and I become irritated when they don't respond the way I expect them to. Unfortunately, my employees are not telepathic and can't read my mind, which can lead to frustration for everyone.

An effective boss should tell an employee specifically what she or he expects, and when they expect it done, and then encourage the employee to ask for assistance or advice if they have any questions or concerns. No one is perfect and it will be easier to build a stronger team if you focus on strengths and not weaknesses. Not every hearing health care provider is made to be a salesperson, a counselor, or a boss. Some may make wonderful clinicians but are incapable of managing employees.

Tech companies have come up with a lot of great tricks to boost their employees' creativity. From having Lady Gaga talk to employees to giving staff year-long sabbaticals, companies are coming up with new and innovative ways to encourage creativity among their employees. Google gives engineers regular time away from their daily jobs to work on creative projects, allowing up to 20% of their workweek to be applied to these projects. The most famous example of a Google service that came out of a "20 percent project," as Google calls them, is Gmail. Nurturing creativity in your workforce can lead to new, innovative ideas for business and happier employees.

In my practice, we have measurable goals and make certain every member of the team has a role in reaching those goals. These goals aren't just sales objectives, but include goals of improving patient satisfaction and reducing the number of patients who seldom wear their hearing aids. Every employee knows and understands their performance is important and critical to the success of the organization. When we reach our goals, we celebrate by giving bonuses, going out to dinner, or getting a day off. I also have fun planning Employee Appreciation Days. These are usually unexpected events that reward employees for jobs well done. Recently, my employees went on a scavenger hunt to earn prizes and then a limo whisked them to lunch and an afternoon of shopping. Other activities have included going to concerts, spas, bowling, and spinning a Wheel of Fortune for prizes.

When things don't go well and the team doesn't reach its goal, we put our heads together and share ideas on what went wrong. Everyone wins when the team works together to make patients happy. Although we would like to believe employees will do what is expected of them and even more, this often doesn't happen. Most hearing health care providers have no formal training in employee management and are so busy seeing patients that they think of employee management as an extra burden. We avoid daily managing the way a lot of people avoid daily exercise and manage only when the situation becomes critical. As a result, employees can get out of shape, and it's not until problems get out of control that we spring into action. If we want employees to "stay in shape" we have to manage them regularly. Daily management doesn't necessarily mean micromanaging; it just means giving employees feedback on a regular basis so they know if their job performance is meeting expectations.

Many managers hesitate to tell employees how to do their jobs because they don't want to give orders. But that's exactly what a boss is supposed to do. The first step in becoming an effective manager is creating structure in the workplace. Employees need written and detailed job descriptions that delineate the duties, responsibilities, and reporting relationships of a particular job. These are necessary so that employees understand exactly what their employer wants them to do.

An employee's performance has to be measured by what is necessary to run an effective and profitable business, not by what the employee *likes* to do. Many times, employees gravitate toward certain tasks or do not complete a task because they really aren't certain what is expected of them or how their employer wants the job done. It's important to give employees regular feedback that includes the positives as well as the negatives. At least yearly reviews of employees should be completed each year to maintain a reliable and stable work force.

A written job description is the first step in the management process, but it must be accompanied by the outcome you will use to determine if the job is being completed successfully. As a follow-up to the written job description, you must determine, in advance, the consequences if the job is not completed satisfactorily. When an employee fails to adhere to the job description, your feedback should be specific. Effective feedback should be focused on a specific behavior. When employees don't meet deadlines or follow written policies, you need to enforce consequences for a job done poorly. Unacceptable behavior that goes unchallenged will be repeated.

When it's necessary to remind employees of their job description, it may be helpful to start the conversation with a compliment. For example, "You did a great job with the reports, but they were a week late. In the future, I expect them to be completed and turned in on time." You want good employees to know they are appreciated, but at the same time you want them to know that failing to follow written protocol is not an option if they want to keep their job.

Management experts report that bosses who involve employees in setting goals and expectations find that employees understand expectations better, are more confident that they can achieve those expectations, and perform at a higher level. If you recognize employees for their accomplishments and support them when they are experiencing difficulty reaching their goals, it is more likely they will be committed to their work. That requires a check-in with them on a regular basis. One of the best ways to monitor an employee's performance is to observe them while they are on the job. Listening to the way a receptionist answers the phone or how an audiologist interacts with a patient can tell more about an employee's performance than a bunch of surveys ever will.

Just because employees know what to do doesn't mean they will do it. If you hear or see something that doesn't live up to your standards, take the employee aside and explain how you expect the situation to be handled in the future. Solve small problems before they become big. No one likes confrontations with employees. Therefore, it's tempting not to bring up small problems with employees, like leaving a patient on hold for five minutes. But remember as the saying goes, "There is no such thing as a small problem." No problem is so small it should be ignored, because small problems fester and become big problems. If you talk to employees about the details of their work on a regular basis, then talking about small problems should be routine and not uncomfortable or confrontational.

As business owners and managers, we need to accept the responsibility of being the boss and act accordingly. An undisciplined workplace is not a healthy environment for employees or managers. Take control today. As long as you are the boss, you might as well be a good one!

Handling a Problematic Employee Situation

If you stay in business long enough, and if you hold employees accountable for their performance, it is inevitable that one day you will have to dismiss an employee. It is never an easy task, but when it's necessary to terminate someone, it's been my experience that the sooner you do it, the better. I recently had the unpleasant experience of dealing with a problem employee. The situation deteriorated over several months and the employee's behavior was affecting everyone in the organization. Despite both verbal and written warnings, it became clear that no amount of effort or explanation was going to rehabilitate this staff member. One might think that a problem employee would recognize that he or she was on the bubble and make the necessary changes to maintain employment, yet that doesn't usually happen.

In my situation, the evidence for dismissal was overwhelming and yet I found myself making every excuse in the book not to fire her. When I received a written complaint from a patient, I knew what I had to do, but a small part of me still wondered whether I had been completely fair with the employee. By the time I had the discussion with the employee about the complaint, the work environment had become a hostile one as her behavior was negatively affecting everyone in the practice.

Being fair is one thing but ignoring problematic behavior is simply irresponsible. Generally speaking, problem employees fall into two categories: those with a bad attitude and those who don't have the skills to do the job properly. Regardless of which category an employee falls into, the first step is to approach the employee to alert them that there is a problem. Although the problem may be obvious to you, the employee may be unaware of it and may be very willing to change their behavior to improve job performance.

All of us, when faced with a stressful situation, experience one of two physiological reactions, fight or flight. Keep this in mind when discussing performance with an employee. You want the initial meeting with the problem employee to be as nonconfrontational as possible. If discussing the problem doesn't help, you have three choices: retrain, discipline, or dismiss.

The first step in the retraining process is to identify the employee's weaknesses and how they relate to job performance. Does the employee lack the skills to accomplish the job to your satisfaction? Is the problem lack of motivation or does the employee need additional training to handle the job? Skills-based performance problems can typically be addressed by training and coaching. Once you have identified the specific weaknesses, you can form a plan that details very specific actions that the employee must take to retain employment. The award for retraining can be a happy employee who is motivated because she or he understands how to be successful.

Behavior problems can rarely be fixed by training. These situations should be handled quickly, explaining the violations and outlining expectations for remediation. You must make it perfectly clear that if the behavior continues, disciplinary action will be taken and if improvements aren't noted, the employee will be terminated. Most importantly, if further violations occur, you have to back up the statement with action. If you allow the unacceptable behavior to continue, you are sending a message to the employee and to the rest of your staff that you will tolerate bad behavior. This is a great way to lose control of your employees.

When you are faced with a serious offense or an employee who has a perpetual bad attitude, you may have no other recourse but to dismiss this person. As long as you are paying people a fair wage and providing a good work environment, there is no reason you should have to endure behavior that could put your business or organization in jeopardy. There are employees who are not well suited for their particular jobs and cannot master the necessary skills, or those who simply refuse to do so. These types of situations bring a business owner or supervisor face-to-face with the need to eliminate a problem they cannot solve any other way.

Before dismissing an employee, you should make certain your legal bases are covered. Background documentation should include the reasons for dismissal and specific examples and dates of any discussions with the employee. State and federal laws prohibit firing workers for reasons such as race or religion, because the worker took family leave, or because the worker complained of illegal company activity. This means you cannot fire an employee without "good cause." However, as the rules and regulations regarding employment are complex, it is wise to seek professional assistance when there is any doubt that termination is justified.

Delivering Extraordinary Service

In today's economy, customer service can be the tool that keeps patients coming back to a practice. A focus on customer service includes answering the phone in a pleasant, upbeat voice. Remember, it's not what you say but how you say it. We have small mirrors near every phone in the office and encourage staff to look and smile before they answer the phone. I have read that when a person smiles while talking on the phone, they are perceived as being friendly. Take the necessary time to thoroughly answer a patient's questions. Make every effort not to put a patient on hold for any extended period of time. If you expect to be tied up for more than a minute, ask the patient if it's acceptable to call him or her back at a designated time and then make certain to fulfill that promise.

It may be my imagination, but it seems that patients are more demanding than ever. Some days I wonder how much further I may have to bend to make people happy. At the end of one particularly challenging day, I breathed a sigh of relief as my final patient walked through the door. It seemed that it had been a day of chronic complainers. When I asked this patient how he was doing, meaning with his new hearing aids not his life, he replied, "These are the days that try men's souls," and proceeded to relay every imaginable problem in his life, his business, his body (trust me when I say that you don't want to know about that one), his crazy mother-in-law, his OCD neighbor, and more. When I finally was able to bring the conversation around to his hearing aids, forty minutes had passed. I was now late for a meeting and really didn't care that his new hearing aids just "didn't work."

When you work with all types and ages of patients, days like this are unavoidable. It is unrealistic to expect to solve every patient's needs, wants, and expectations. However, we must respond to every concern a patient expresses. A less than satisfied patient will look elsewhere for a provider. Actually, when a patient complains about a product or service received, it can be a blessing in disguise. We all know that a happy patient tells almost no one and an unhappy patient tells everyone so dissatisfied patients can have a dramatic impact on the success of a business. Because competitors are offering the same services and products you are, it will be the satisfied patients who bring in repeat business, as well as new patients. Therefore, resolving complaints in a quick and complete manner is essential to maintaining a successful business.

Your patient's problem might be entirely out of your hands. On the other hand, you could have made an honest mistake.

Either way, offering an apology helps bring down a person's defenses. Once you calm the patient, remind them that you care. Whether you are responsible for the complaint or not, be aware that any bad experience can lead to resentment and lost business. Let the patient know you are sorry they are unhappy and that you will do whatever you can to resolve the issue. Whatever you do, don't get angry. It's impossible to win an argument with an angry person. Reinforce what you are going to do to correct the unfortunate situation, and even if the patient is at fault, don't remind them of that.

When complaints do occur, deal with them immediately and resolve them completely. It doesn't matter whether you feel you are at fault or not. The only thing that matters is that the patient is satisfied that you have done everything possible to resolve their concern. Resolution may require refunding money, exchanging a product, or doing a complimentary repair. It's imperative to make sure the patient is completely satisfied with the outcome. I don't know about you, but I can't read minds. Don't assume you know what the patient expects, just ask them. Exceeding a patient's expectations is the best way to convert an unhappy patient into a raving fan of the business.

It is human nature to become defensive when faced with a complaint. Staff members will naturally react this way unless you train them to react differently. When confronted by an angry patient, the challenge is to resist becoming defensive and to approach the situation calmly and professionally. Tell the front office staff how you would like them to handle a difficult situation and help them to understand why patients get angry. The patient may also have other issues besides the frustration that accompanies a hearing problem. A staff member on the front lines must have the authority to handle some complaints when they happen in order to make the patient happy. Don't waste a patient's time keeping him waiting "to speak to the boss." That may only exacerbate the situation.

Every business relies on repeat business to grow, so it doesn't make good business sense not to use customer complaints to improve. When mistakes happen, take time to discuss them with your employees and ask how things could be handled differently in the future. Many complaints are not a result of a mistake, but rather misreading a patient's expectations or needs.

Although you can't take every complaint to heart, take note of each one to determine if there is a "common denominator" that could be changed. What if the patient has no basis for the complaint? You could argue the point but most of the time, it's easier to take a deep breath and ask the patient what he or she would like you to do. It is not who "wins" but how you end the game. Although it is important to try to satisfy every patient, there are some patients who simply can't be satisfied and it is in the best interest of the business to let those patients find another service provider. I have only "fired" three patients in all my years in business, and two begged to come back.

For every formal complaint, there may be ten or more other patients who were dissatisfied and felt like complaining, but never did. Instead, they switched service providers and told all their friends of their dissatisfaction. When a patient complains, it means that person cares enough to give you a second chance, so the next time a patient shares a frustration or concern, embrace this feedback instead of dreading, denying, or resenting it. People often give more weight to the negative. It has been reported that an unhappy patient will share their feelings with five times more people than a happy patient. Because patients widely broadcast their views in person and online, every interaction is critical to maintaining a good relationship with patients, and these relationships are key to maintaining a successful practice. Therefore, if you wonder how far you have to bend for your patients, the answer is as far as it takes to make and keep them happy.

Staying Connected to Patient Base

I recently went through my electronic patient records in an attempt to uncover patients we had lost touch with, and then I was determined to devise a way to get them back. It was a very painful investigation! I was sad to see the number of patients with whom we had lost touch or that had changed to another provider. This is especially troubling because it is costing more and more to attract new patients through marketing activities. A practice simply can't afford to throw away patients. People are living longer, and attracting new patients is increasingly more expensive, so we have to make every effort to retain current patients and to turn them into "patients for life."

A common business maxim that gets thrown around is that it costs 5 to 10 times more to get a new patient than to keep an existing one, and yet we often spend our time, energy, and money marketing and advertising to get new patients to fill the gaps in the schedule. Consider exploring the numbers of patients leaving the practice, and then investigate the reasons why and devise a plan to recapture some of them. It's inevitable that some patients will leave, but it's important to the health of the business to correct any problems that may be causing patients to leave.

Most patients who leave, do so quietly and without warning. Take an hour or two and check how many of your current patients haven't been seen in the past year and then contact them to let them know you noticed and that you would like them to return to the practice for their hearing help.

Patients would like to understand the condition of their hearing, but too often, we are so impressed by what we know that we use way too much technical jargon when explaining hearing loss and options for rehabilitation. The jargon does little to shed light on the real problem and will often do nothing but confuse a patient. Patients will be far more likely to understand their situations and trust proposed solutions if and when they understand the problem. There is nothing better for a long-term patient-provider relationship than making sure the patient feels you are listening to their every word (that is difficult with some). It's extremely important that patients feel their provider is focused on their problems, and is taking adequate time to explain any and all possible solutions.

Our patients may like us, may think our service is good, and our practice is fine in every regard, but still may change providers if they can't schedule a convenient time to come for an appointment. Everyone leads busy lives these days, and lack of flexibility and availability can cause patients to look elsewhere, especially in a situation when they need service. Promote telehealth access to the practice as a means of offering easy access to the hearing health care. We encourage patients to call between 10 AM to 11 AM and 2 PM to 3 PM for telehealth access to professionals.

Although we want to treat every patient well, there are definitely some patients who deserve special treatment. Identify the patients who have been the most supportive and invested the most money with you (not so hard with electronic records) and consider offering them special treatment, such as executive hours, no charge service on certain items, extended payment plans, and/or trials on new products before they are released to the public.

Scheduling Effectively

Scheduling for maximum efficiency should be the goal of any practice. When it comes to business, efficiency is crucial and an essential element of profitability. Most hearing health care practices employ one professional and one support person. I would recommend that the professional concentrate their energy on producing revenue, and delegate to the support personnel tasks that don't require the education and expertise of a professional, such as completing paperwork, cleaning and repairing hearing aids, and ordering supplies.

CareCredit recently completed some research that suggests that Baby Boomers entering the market today prefer fewer appointments than their older counterparts. Therefore, it may be more efficient to schedule a longer initial appointment so that there is time to complete a hearing aid fitting if the evaluation indicates that amplification is needed. In my practice, demonstrating technology and better hearing is always a part of the initial evaluation when a hearing loss is identified. If you maintain a small stock of RIC aids, it can be easy and efficient to demonstrate appropriate aids, and then proceed with the fitting if the patient agrees to purchase amplification. A word of caution here that a patient should also pay for the aids when leaving with them. I know many colleagues that allow patients to "try" hearing aids for a week or two before they pay for them, but I don't recommend that for *many* reasons. Primarily, because if we as professionals diagnose a hearing problem and the patient needs and can benefit from aids, why should they *try* and not *buy*? Personally, it's been my experience that patients expect to pay for aids if they leave with them. Collecting payment in full at the time of fitting is the best way to avoid cash flow problems.

Using Support Personnel

While completing my AuD degree, I conducted a time study of the types of activities audiologists in various types of practice settings perform on a daily basis. Data revealed the audiologists spent more than one-third, and probably closer to one-half, of their workdays performing minor, time-consuming tasks that could have been performed by lesser qualified individuals. It would seem that delegating those tasks to support personnel would allow professionals to see more patients, potentially generating more revenue, which logically could lead to an increase in profitability. Most other medical professions (physicians, nurses, optometrists, dentists, veterinarians) and allied health professions (physical therapists, occupational therapists) have well-developed technician positions. Just imagine how many more patients you could see if you didn't have to clean hearing aids, complete order and repair forms, set up testing procedures, troubleshoot equipment, teach patients how to clean, insert, and remove hearing aids. Not to mention demonstrating how to use remote controls, wireless accessories, t-coils, rehab programs, loop systems, and other assistive devices. With this type of assistance, the professional can spend more time providing patients with vitally needed services, such as family counseling, outlining realistic expectations, performing speech in noise testing, or assessing central processing function.

The use of support personnel in hearing health care practices is still considered by some to be controversial despite the fact that the concept has been endorsed by every professional hearing health care organization for the past forty years! With the burgeoning need for hearing health care services, and a potential shortage of qualified professionals, the best way to increase productivity and profitability of a business may be to hire support personnel. I have heard rumblings from colleagues that their state license will not allow them to use support personnel. In fact, I have found just the opposite to be true.

I was forced to add an Audiology Assistant to my practice many years ago. The steady growth of the practice and the lack of audiologists in the small community in which my business is located necessitated the need to hire support personnel to

---

Example of a Job Description for an Audiology Assistant

Reports to: President/ Operations Manager

Job Summary: Responsible for rendering professional patient care within the practice in support of Audiology and professional staff

Responsibilities include but are not limited to: Managing the service department, satisfactorily making earmold impressions when requested by professionals (this task must be allowed in state licensure law), modification of earmolds and hearing aid casings, performing minor hearing aid repairs, completing order forms for new hearing aids and earmolds, stocking treatment rooms with supplies, and supporting professionals in the care of patients. This employee will be required to submit monthly performance reports to Operations Manager. In addition to above, complete notes section of Sycle must be completed following by the end of the business day when the appointment occurred.

---

perform tasks that did not require the education and expertise of an audiologist. However, as the practice continued to grow, it became evident that the use of support personnel improved productivity, service accessibility, quality of patient care, and patient satisfaction. Although the concept of using support personnel is not widespread, a review of practices today indicate that support personnel are being used successfully in a variety of practice settings, including the military, the VA, educational institutions, hospitals, industrial settings, and private practices. In fact, using support personnel can provide valuable assistance to professionals by increasing patient contact hours, reducing wait time and improving patient satisfaction.

The hearing health care professional must maintain clinical and legal responsibility over the support personnel, and is morally responsible for these individuals, as the duties that the assistant is allowed to perform are regulated by state licensure laws. The hearing health care professional must also ensure that good quality of patient care is maintained. Adequate and continual training is also essential. The tasks of record-keeping, assisting in clinical research, clerical duties, such as completing all paperwork, and other administrative support functions can also be delegated to an assistant.

The time for using support personnel in hearing health care practices has arrived and, in fact, is long overdue. Using our time to focus on activities that best utilize our education and expertise, and delegating lesser tasks, can be a big step toward increasing the profitability of a hearing health care business.

7

Getting Patients to Commit to Better Hearing

You may dread having to tell a patient that you diagnosed a hearing problem and then have to suggest that to get assistance for the problem will require the patient to purchase a plan that could cost thousands of dollars. Most patients aren't going to jump up and down and say, "That's awesome news" or "Oh boy, I can't wait to spend what I consider to be 'lots' of money to get the help you suggest that I need." The most common response, when you explain the test results and suggest that the patient could benefit from hearing help in the form of hearing aid, is that the solution costs too much money. Unfortunately, many patients we see won't actually *want* the help we recommend. However, because 90+% of patients with hearing loss have sensory loss, the only way to actually *help a patient* is to convince them to get hearing aids. Objections are very common in any "sales" process, and if you are recommending something that costs money, it is indeed a sales process, regardless of the profession or vocation, so we shouldn't be surprised or blindsided by them. We should, in fact, expect objections to better hearing when it involves purchasing something.

According to industry statistics, the average "Help Rate" of a hearing health care professional is less than 50%. This doesn't seem to disturb most people, but it really concerns me. If someone takes the step to make an appointment to confirm what they already feel is a problem, and a hearing loss is diagnosed, isn't it our responsibility as professionals to convince the patient to get help? Maybe I am different than most, but I don't make an appointment with a health professional unless I feel there is a problem and I *know* I need help. So if industry numbers hold true and only 50% of patients that visit a hearing health care professional are getting the help they need in the form of hearing aids, shouldn't we work harder and get better at responding to these objections that we hear every day from patients?

The real problem may be that most hearing health care professionals were never taught how to respond to these common objections. Developing better ways to respond will take time and practice, but the end result will be worth the effort and the satisfaction of helping more patients hear better should be reason enough to improve at sharing information in a way that convinces more patients to proceed with hearing aids. I'm sure all of us have experienced a patient who said that they did not want to wear hearing aids, but once they got them and acclimated to them, they were happy they took the advice to heart and commented that better hearing was well worth the cost.

The concept of selling hearing technology to patients isn't always a comfortable one, which is not surprising, as most hearing health care professionals aren't taught how to do that in our coursework and training. I would contend that learning how to persuade patients to get help for their problem is one of the most important things we do. Presenting information on hearing enhancement in a manner that is convincing is actually not about selling something. It's about getting acquainted with a patient; learning their hearing and communicative deficiencies and then agreeing on a solution that best suits those needs. The consequences of doing a poor job of convincing a patient to obtain help can result in social isolation and deterioration of quality of life, not to mention the cognitive decline that recent research suggests. From this perspective, it seems not only our professional responsibility to *sell* our solutions, but our duty to do everything we can to be very good at it. It doesn't take a mathematician to realize that helping more patients to hear better isn't just good for patients; it is also good for business.

The first step to improving the process of convincing a patient to get help for their hearing loss is tracking appointment outcomes. Many of us think we help more patients than we actually do. Most practice management software includes some form of tracking. If this option is not available to you, start a spreadsheet and keep track of how many patients you see who are candidates for amplification and then record how many patients you actually convince to purchase them. The tracking should include new patients, and also current patients who have aids over three or four years old, or those patients who are not hearing well with their present hearing aids that could benefit from new technology. If you participate in third-party reimbursement programs such as Medicaid, do not include those patients in the tracking process as you really don't have to convince them because payment is not required and adding these individuals to the tracking can skew results and make it appear that you are convincing more patients than you actually are.

Diagnosing a hearing loss is just the first step in helping a patient. Convincing patients to obtain help in the form of hearing aids directly relates to the ability to persuade them that *now* is the time to take the step to do something about their problem. I find it helpful to take some time during the initial interview to learn what motivated the patient to make an appointment before I test their hearing. It's been my experience that it is possible to assess motivation and actually gain a patient's commitment to better hearing even before beginning the evaluation. For instance, after spending time discussing a patient's motivation for making the appointment and how the deterioration of hearing ability may be affecting their life, you might say, "Mrs. Jones, you indicated that you are having difficulty hearing your grandchildren and you no longer enjoy going out socially because you can't understand conversations. If I can help you hear better in those situations, is that the help you are looking for today?"

Discovering a patient's motivation for making the appointment is a key element in convincing them to take the step of investing in better hearing. There is a *specific* reason that the patient made the appointment at that day and time. I'm sure they have seen many of your advertisements, and have missed out on conversations at social gatherings many times before, but something happened that caused that patient to make an appointment that day. Uncovering that salient event is key in helping motivate them to take action for a problem that is certain to have been affecting their life for a significant period of time.

Do not become discouraged or alarmed if a patient objects before, during, or after you recommend hearing aids. In fact, we should expect objections. Objections are nothing more than comments or concerns that require clarification. An objection doesn't necessarily mean the patient does not agree with the diagnosis or doesn't want to work with you to achieve a solution. Patient opposition may be nothing more than a request for more time to make a decision, or a need for clarification. There is a big difference between an excuse and an objection. Most importantly, don't be intimidated by objections. Rather, step back and let the patient express concerns and then address them one at a time. A "No" or "I want to think about it" may mean that you haven't gotten to the real heart of the problem of what brought the patient to you in the first place. The patient may just need more information before proceeding.

Developing an Effective Presentation

One of the crucial elements in convincing patients to take our advice is developing a detailed, well-thought-out process for testing and presenting information to patients. Used consistently, this process should become routine and comfortable.

The initial patient interview represents the discovery phase of the appointment. It is important to understand the decisions a patient needs to make to progress toward the goal of obtaining help for a hearing problem. This requires mutual understanding every step of the way. If at any point, there is not a mutual decision to move forward, the desired result of helping a patient hear better will not be achieved. This process should be smooth, friendly, and nonthreatening, thus making the patient feel comfortable. The goal of the initial interview should be to identify the salient event that caused the patient to finally make the appointment. An example of an initial interview may be something like this:

> **Professional**—"Good day, Mr. Duensing. My name
> is Dr. Kasewurm and I am going to evaluate your
> hearing today. Let me give you a brief tour of the

office, get you a cup of coffee, and then we can sit down and chat to see what brings you here today." We then take a brief walk around the office and sit down together in a quiet room.

Professional—"It is so nice to meet you Mr. Duensing. Can you share with me why you came for a hearing evaluation today?"

Patient—"I saw your advertisement on Facebook."

Professional—"We have been running Facebook ads for some time and we have been in business for many years. This isn't the first time you have seen one of our ads, is it Mr. Duensing?" Patient shakes his head indicating "No."

Professional—"Then, I am curious as to why you made *this* appointment and what concerns you may have about your hearing."

Discovering a patient's motivation for making an appointment is a key element in convincing them to take action and to embrace the idea of investing in better hearing. During this process it is important to ask questions, paraphrase the patient's responses, acknowledge their viewpoint, listening intently and looking them in the eye. This type of dialogue will hopefully uncover the significant event that led the patient to make the appointment. Although most patients have known a problem existed for some time, it usually takes a specific incident or remark to get them to finally make an appointment to investigate the problem.

Before beginning the evaluation, explain to the patient what to expect during the testing process. Remember, many clinicians use the term *hearing test* and that can imply that a patient's concentration or effort can somehow affect the outcome. Attempt to put patients at ease. Ask if they have any questions and assure them that all they have to do is relax, listen, and respond. An example of this could be:

Professional—"Mr. Duensing, I will begin the evaluation by looking in your ear canal to make certain there is no debris that could affect the results and will remove it if necessary. Then I will evaluate your hearing to see how well you are able to hear various different pitches of sound. After I have completed that process, I will have you listen to words to see how well you are able to understand voices when they are loud enough. Because the majority of people with hearing loss have difficulty understanding in noisy situations, I will also evaluate your ability to hear in background noise. Initial speech testing is designed to assess your *potential* for understanding when speech is loud enough to hear well, which means it may be louder than an average voice. Once that testing has been completed, I will assess your ability to understand speech at a normal loudness level. If a hearing deficit is identified, I will determine a prescription for better hearing and will actually demonstrate how you *should* be hearing. Hearing loss occurs very gradually and most people are unaware of what they miss. At that time, I will use your spouse's voice (or whoever accompanied them to the appointment) in the testing process. Does this sound OK to you? Do you have any questions about the testing process?"

After completing testing and demonstrating the potential with appropriately programmed hearing aids placed on their ears, I sit with the patient and the third party that is with them and then present the audiometric results. How much time have you actually spent on presenting hearing test results in a manner that is clear, concise, and effective? Often, the information is much too long and detailed and the patient's eyes glass over as we share particulars of inner ear stereocilia and their ability to transform the mechanical energy of sound into electrical signals, which ultimately leads to an excitation of the auditory nerve. I am obviously being facetious, but it's critical to record and then analyze how you describe test results to patients to make certain that the explanation is simple and easy to understand and then include a strong recommendation of your proposed solution to the problem that you identified. Having a third party present at the appointment dramatically increases the likelihood that the patient will choose to take action for their problem at the time of the visit. The person making appointments should inform the patient of the need to bring someone along to their hearing evaluation when the appointment is made. The patient should again be reminded of that need when the appointment is confirmed. This isn't something that should be left to chance. A script to follow should be available, and the inclusion of third parties should be tracked on a monthly basis. An example of such a script could be:

> "In order for Dr. Kasewurm to effectively test and access your hearing, she will use a familiar voice during the evaluation. Therefore, she would like you to bring a friend or family member to the appointment for this purpose. Whom will you be able to bring to this appointment?"

I know this may seem archaic to some, but the truth is that we are assessing more than just hearing. The evaluation involves communication and that takes two people, not to mention that many people are unlikely to make a decision on their own without consulting another party. Having a significant other or family member involved in the assessment will increase the likelihood of the patient making a decision at the time of the appointment. Although we don't want to ever force someone to take action, the patient usually has waited a considerable amount of time before making the appointment, and the time to get them to take action is *NOW*, or they may continue to live affected by the devastating effects of hearing loss for a much longer period of time.

Dealing with Common Objections

Many hearing health care professionals are intimidated by the concept of selling, but the fact is that the majority of patients that visit our offices suffer with sensory hearing loss, and the only way we can help them is to convince them to do something about their hearing loss and that usually involves obtaining hearing aids. On a basic level, selling is simply listening and understanding what a patient wants and needs to do to take action. I have always believed that promoting better hearing is like religion—if you believe it, it won't be difficult to get patients to believe it too.

What follows are some suggestions on how to handle the five most common objections that we hear from patients every day.

Objection—My Hearing Isn't Bad Enough

The objection that hearing isn't bad enough to get help is one of the easiest to deal with, as we can show the patient what they miss by doing testing at a normal listening level instead of at an optimal level. We can demonstrate the potential for better hearing by placing appropriately programmed hearing aids on their ears as they listen to recorded speech or discourse from a third person that has accompanied them. When a patient shares this objection, perhaps what they are actually saying is that they are not convinced their problem is severe enough to spend a significant amount money and time to get hearing aids. In this situation, think back to the case history and the original reason the patient made the appointment. It's also important to *show* patients what they are missing. I usually explain to the patient that the testing in the booth determines potential for understanding speech because the volume has been increased to maximize abilities to understand when speech is loud enough. Testing performed at a normal loudness level (40 to 45 dB HTL) will reveal how well a patient is actually able to hear and understand in a real-life situation. After completing unaided discrimination tests presented at a normal listening level, I find this to be the perfect time to demonstrate amplification to show patients what they are missing by not wearing hearing aids.

Objection—I Want to Think About It

Many people do not like to make on-the-spot decisions. However, if a patient is convinced of the need for help and the benefits of remediation, they are likely to take action. When a patient objects to the recommendation to get hearing aids, they may have questions about benefit. One response might be, "Mr. Jones, obviously I would like you to get the help you need. Is there some information that I can give you today that would help you make your decision? The reason I ask is that I want to make sure that I have explained everything to you and answered any questions you may have. This hearing loss did not happen overnight and is not going to get any better if you wait. I would like to get you over the hurdle and get this started today by taking some impressions so we can get the process started." Or, on a lighter note, "You told me you have noticed this problem for the past five years. How much longer do you need to think about it?"

Objection—I Can't Afford It

This may or may not be a legitimate objection. The real question is whether the patient actually doesn't have the money to make the purchase, whether they don't feel the amplification is worth the money, or whether they just don't want to spend the money. Many of us can recall at least one patient who didn't *look* like he could afford help and said he *couldn't* afford help only to discover the person was a multimillionaire. I can give many personal accounts of patients who said they couldn't afford help and then went to a less qualified and more expensive competitor who was able to convince them to purchase aids. Never, and I do mean *never,* judge a person's ability to consume. Every patient deserves to hear better and it is our responsibility as professionals to recommend what we feel is *best* for a patient and then let the patient decide about affordability. Although there are some patients who truly don't have the money to purchase hearing aids, it's been my experience that many patients who visit our offices already know what hearing aids cost because they have been referred by another patient who already shared information on pricing. Just like the other objections, we can't be surprised by them and need to work at discovering better ways to handle them.

Objection—I Need to Talk with My Spouse or Loved One

Most patients won't make a purchase decision of such magnitude without discussing it with a spouse. However, the spouse probably knew of the appointment and, in fact, even encouraged the visit. In this scenario, the first option is to suggest that the spouse or significant other accompany the patient when the appointment is made. I have read that patients are 80% more likely to take action when an influencer comes to the appointment with them. If the patient comes alone, you may say, "I have identified a significant hearing problem in our testing, Mr. Jones. Obviously, this is affecting communication between you and your spouse so I would like to make another appointment when your spouse can accompany you so we can discuss this problem together."

Objection — Hearing Aids Don't Work

Many of us have heard a patient refer to someone who has aids that sit in a drawer unused. In this case, it is best not to try to disprove why the friend doesn't like their hearing aids, but rather to say, "It is true that there are patients who don't wear their hearing aids, but in your situation . . . " Don't spend a great deal of time trying to disprove a claim that you know nothing about, but rather spend your time on the issues that make your patient an excellent candidate for help, and why you believe it is in their best interest to proceed with the steps to improve their hearing.

The most important point is not to run and retreat at the patient's first "No." Try to determine what is actually holding the patient back and return to the reasons the patient made the appointment in the first place—missing important information at work, feeling left out of conversations with loved ones, or avoiding social situations. Never try to manipulate a patient into taking action. You may get them to take action in the short run, but in the long run, the patient may return the aids or let them sit in a drawer.

Remember, a patient's "No" might be definite for now, but it may not remain so forever. When a patient objects to a recommendation, don't take it personally. Rejection is an unavoidable part of working with all types of personalities when trying to help them with hearing problems, and there will be some patients that are easier to connect with than others. People who have lived with hearing loss may have a difficult time understanding what it will be like to hear well again. Too often, we tell patients what they should do, but we don't show them what it would be like to hear well. Demonstrating the latest technology and showing a patient how hearing aids can improve the ability to hear conversational speech can be a very effective way to convince them to take action.

Objections can be minimized by having the right combination of trust and professionalism. The major reason objections arise at the end of the presentation is because concerns weren't effectively addressed, or perhaps the patient just isn't ready to proceed with better hearing. However, I find that with more investigation, this isn't usually the case. It's not unusual for people to be indecisive when making decisions that have a significant impact on their lives, but we can't give up on a patient just because "No" is their initial reaction to our recommendation. No one really wants to have a hearing loss, but help, in the form of hearing aids, can be just what they want once they understand the consequences of doing nothing.

To Try or Not to Try?

I am going to open what always seems to be a "can of worms" when I give presentations, and that is the topic of *Free Trials*. I have never been a fan of "try before you buy" offers. It's been my experience that trials may be free to a patient, but are anything but free for a business. A patient who has nothing invested won't hesitate to waste your time. However, many colleagues disagree with my theory and contend that trials work in their practices. A few colleagues, who put **all** of their aids out on trial, with no money down before recommending that a patient purchase the aids, claim that 90% to 95% of patients who take the aids on trial purchase them.

I received so much pushback on this topic when I challenged the validity of trials in a recent presentation that I decided to retest the concept in my own practice. My staff and I set up several trial groups for patients: Group A consisted of patients who had been evaluated at the office, diagnosed with a hearing loss, and didn't purchase aids at the time of the visit (TNS); Group B consisted of current patients who had been wearing their current set of hearing aids for four years or more. We offered each of these groups the opportunity to wear new technology for a period of one to two weeks with no money invested up front.

Both groups of patients in the trials yielded similar results, and 86% indicated that they did indeed hear and communicate better with the new aids. However, 60% of patients who tried the aids, and had no money invested, returned them, and did not purchase the aids. This number is actually consistent with industry averages and with my previous experiences with trials in my practice. The goal in my practice is to convince at least 80% of patients who need aids (including mild high frequency losses), and patients with aids over 4 years old, to obtain help in the form of hearing aids. This goal is ambitious and not easy to achieve but we work at it and regularly review our protocols and what we say to patients if we aren't reaching our goal. This is a robust goal even for myself despite my thirty plus years of experience. I believe that if better hearing and amplification is the best outcome for a patient, then we owe it to patients to do our best to convince them to move forward with amplification. It's been my experience and the experience of other colleagues that patients who don't commit to better hearing at the time of their initial appointment don't come back to us, but often purchase from a competitor within a short period of time following their initial evaluation.

I can hear the skeptics out there. *"Dr. Gyl doesn't know what she is talking about. Trials work!"* However, most practitioners don't have the numbers to back these claims up, as tracking isn't commonplace in our industry. All I can say is, "Show me the numbers!" I will believe it when I see the numbers. And make sure the trials are all based on the same definition of candidacy. It's easy to tweak the numbers to improve the outcome. I don't want to hear, "I think __% purchased," and I hear that often. It's human nature to imagine outcomes better than they actually are. Track your numbers on trials and also track how many "no charge" visits you invest in those trials. Time is money. I hear so much chatter that we have to charge and get paid for what we do, and I agree, but trials and "no charge" visits are also giving away expertise and services and are very costly to a business.

8

Financial Aspects
of a Practice

The Pricing Conundrum

Pricing is a controversial topic and yet it's an essential one because establishing an appropriate pricing structure can literally make or break a business. The conundrum is how to price products and services so they are not too expensive and not too cheap. Although there are many ways to formulate a pricing structure, the one that's most appropriate for you is the one that will make money for your practice. I could make an argument for charging more in my practice because I have four full-time assistants who repair hearing aids in minutes while the patient waits. You need to be able to make a case for your pricing strategy. If you can't, you need to build one because when a patient looks you in the eye and asks you why you and your organization are worth their money, your answer had better be convincing.

Every business wrestles with the question of how to set prices because there is no magic formula to determine the right price. Before setting prices, you must first understand the market for your product or service, the channels of distribution, your competition, and the cost of operating your business. It's imperative to be keenly aware of all costs and carefully analyze what is involved in those costs. The goal is to find the price at which profit is maximized and demand is not affected. Many hearing health care professionals make the mistake of setting prices based on what their competition is charging. But every business is different, so pricing should be established based on what it costs to run your business.

The biggest mistake that I have seen practice owners make is charging too little. It's easy to get intimidated by price ads run by competitors and then to react with your own price reductions. What we charge isn't about price unless we make it about price. The prices we charge are about value—the value of hearing better and the benefits of working with a professional who has the education, expertise, and the persistence to make certain successful outcomes are achieved. It's about the value of the services that we provide to keep the patient hearing better. Patients certainly are concerned about the cost of hearing aids and want to feel like they are getting good value for their money. But, the fact is, cheaper prices have never translated into more hearing aids being sold.

Regardless of your pricing structure, a patient can always find a provider with cheaper hearing aids, such as the Internet, sporting magazines, eBay, and Costco, just to name a few. But benefits always outweigh price in this industry, so instead of lowering prices, adhere to a best practices protocol. This consists of a comprehensive test battery, including measures of loudness discomfort and speech-in-noise testing, and complete real-ear measurements to ensure that patients are deriving optimal benefit from their hearing aids. If patients understand the value of what we do, if they achieve adequate hearing benefit, and feel they are being treated fairly and courteously, they won't mind paying the prices we charge. Unfortunately, some hearing professionals are uncomfortable with the prices they charge. If patients sense that insecurity, they will also be uncomfortable with the charges and will walk out without getting help for their hearing loss. It's essential that you be able to justify your charges in your own mind before presenting them to patients.

In a successful business, prices should be set to cover total costs, plus some margin of profit. There are two main costs in a hearing health care practice:

- The cost of goods sold, i.e., hearing aids and earmolds.
- The costs of operating the business, called operating expenses. These include owner distributions, marketing, employee salaries, rent, utilities, insurance, and office supplies.

Any time I spend time talking with colleagues or scanning through Facebook groups targeted at hearing healthcare professionals, I see people querying about what to charge for hearing aids and services. Many people are concerned, and I understand why with the competition from big-box stores and the increasing numbers of third-party administrator programs that have emerged and control what we are able to charge. Our margins are shrinking, but our fees can't be dictated by an outside party that knows nothing about what it costs to run our specific business. Pricing strategies have to be established so that profit is adequate to pay expenses. There are several known and typically used pricing strategies that I will attempt to explain below.

Examples of Pricing Strategies

Multiplier of Cost of Goods Sold (COGS)

Some practitioners establish their COGS for a particular time period, and use some multiplier, such as two or three times the COGS, to set their prices. Some business owners may also look at the annual surveys in hearing health care journals to discover the average price that a patient in the United States pays for a hearing aid.

Manufacturer's Suggested Retail Price (MSRP)

Another traditional way to look at prices is to take the manufacturer's retail price schedule and work down. A 50% off MSRP might sound appealing to a patient, but there may be little evidence to determine if the price is reasonable or if it allows for adequate profit for the practice.

Competitive Pricing

Most practitioners know where the top and bottom ends of pricing are in their market and believe that it will be detrimental for their business to price themselves out of the market. Setting prices slightly higher or lower than the competition creates a price structure that has no real figures to back it up. Although this might be a simple strategy, it doesn't establish a consistent pricing policy or insure that costs will be covered and profit will be achieved.

Any of these strategies may prove successful for some business owners. But the most effective way to implement your chosen strategy is to contact a CPA, give them a spreadsheet of your income and expenses, and let them use their expertise to help you establish the most appropriate pricing strategy for the practice.

A Unique Pricing Option

Many of you may have heard me talk about the pricing strategy that is based on Dan Ariely's book, *Predictably Irrational*, which I call Consumer Advantage Pricing. We've used the pricing structure for several years in my practice and it's proven to be very successful for raising the average selling price of our hearing aid technologies.

Here's how **Consumer Advantage Pricing** works. When you have two options, people are forced to make a decision between the two. Consumer Advantage Pricing involves adding a *third* option that is priced *exactly the same* as the more expensive option. Why do smart people make irrational decisions every day? It's often because of the way information is presented. Research has shown that consumers change their preference between two options when also presented with a third option.

Decision making for humans is difficult, so why not make it easier? Sometimes we give too many choices to our patients and they don't know which one to pursue. We explain several different types of hearing aids, mention the option of custom earmolds, and include the option of Bluetooth connectivity, and then let the patient make the decision instead of offering a strong recommendation, which can be very confusing for a patient. By providing a method of comparison, we are more likely to increase the number of patients who will make a decision on the spot, rather than having to go home and think about it.

> In order for this pricing strategy to work, you must offer three choices—no more, no less!

Typical pricing strategy

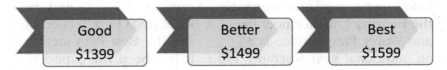

Figure 8–1. Good/Better/Best strategy example, but not actual pricing.

For years, I employed a *Good, Better, Best* type of technology presentation with prices equally spaced apart (Figure 8–1). Although some patients chose the best technology, it was most typical for patients to choose the middle option. Before implementing Consumer Advantage Pricing in my practice, the ASP hadn't increased significantly in almost twenty years. I know some people reading this article are saying, "This will never work for my practice. My patients or my demographic won't support such a concept." I have heard it all before but I have yet to talk to someone who implemented this strategy who hasn't found it beneficial for business.

The objection that I have found to be the most relevant is explaining to patients why the better and the best technologies have the same price. Believe it or not, this isn't a comment that we hear often. Patients just seem to be satisfied that they can obtain "more" for "less." When someone does inquire as to why the better and best products are the same price, we simply respond, "Since our results indicate that patients are more satisfied and perform the best with the best technology, I negotiated a better price with our manufacturers to make it possible for more patients to get what they need."

Let me stress the aspects of this pricing structure that are essential for its success:

- Offer only three prices for your Hearing Enhancement Plan. It's important that it is three pricing levels—no more and no less.
- Raise the price of your BETTER technology and Worry Free Service Plan so it is exactly the SAME as the BEST technology and Worry Free Service Plan, and then add something extra free to the BEST.

- Do not *decrease* the price of the option for the Best plan. *Increase* the price for the Better plan.

For instance, perhaps the Hearing Enhancement Plan for Good technology and Worry Free Service is $_____, and then the Hearing Enhancement Plan for Better AND Best Technology and Worry Free Service is $_____, but the Best Plan included an additional year warranty FREE. It has been my experience and many colleagues have shared their success with me that this type of pricing structure will definitely raise the average selling price of technology in the practice.

Bundling, Unbundling, and Itemizing

The debate over bundling versus unbundling in hearing aid pricing rages on. Although the unbundled method of pricing is seen in a minority of practices, the issue has come front and center because the cost of hearing health care is seen as being too expensive, even by our government, as was confirmed with the recent passage of the Over The Counter Hearing Aid bill.

The most common method of pricing currently is in a bundled, or packaged format, where fees for the hearing aids and those services associated with choosing, fitting, adjusting, and servicing the hearing aids are billed in a single charge for a given period of time. However, with the advent of so many low-cost providers, unbundling has been promoted as a good pricing option in an effort to keep from losing patients to the many low-cost providers of hearing aids.

Itemizing has also become a popular pricing option. There are many ways to incorporate itemization into a pricing strategy. You could choose to present a fee for the device(s) and present a separate fee for the associated professional services. Or, some colleagues present a fee for the hearing aids and then the patient has a choice of different service package options. In this model, the professional is still collecting the fees for the devices and the associated services up front, but the fees are itemized so it is easier for a patient to see what they are paying for. One caution to point out is if an established business has been utilizing a bundled form of pricing, gross revenue will suffer in the first couple of years because the cost for services won't be collected up front, but should be realized in subsequent years. Creating a fee structure that separates the cost of the hearing aid(s) from the services associated with the evaluation, fitting, orientation, delivery, counseling, and long-term care and management of these devices provides the opportunity to highlight the importance of our professional services.

Examples of Pricing Strategies

Bundled model of pricing

Premier Hearing Enhancement Plan $_____

This type of plan usually includes the hearing aids, the fitting, and all service and adjustments for a given period of time.

Unbundled model of pricing

Premier Hearing Enhancement Plan $_____

Pricing is for hearing aids only, and all associated services are billed separately.

Itemized model of pricing

Premier Technology Hearing aids $_____

Premier Service Package included during three-year warranty period

    Fitting and one follow-up visit $_____

    One repair per year for years two and three $_____

    Annual evaluations each year 3 @ $_____

    Three cleanings per year 9 @ $_____

    Batteries for three years $_____

    Wax management twice a year 6 @ $_____

    Reprogramming once a year 3 @ $_____

Total value of Service Package $_____

Total Investment in Better Hearing $_____

So what method is best? The answer to that question has to be based upon the cost to run your particular business or practice. As usual, my advice is to measure and monitor help rates to see what is working with your patients. If help rates decline, then it's necessary to evaluate the reasons patients are not taking your advice, and how much is based upon the objections to the cost of treatment, and then consider a different pricing strategy. In these changing times, it may well take a combination of methods to succeed.

Regardless of the work setting, there will always be some patients that attempt to get out of paying at the time of their visit. An elderly patient of mine needed new hearing aids to be able to hear well at her upcoming 90th birthday party. Unfortunately, the patient did not have the resources to purchase the aids, but her family assured me they could handle the expense if I would agree to 90 days same as cash. Of course I didn't want to be the reason this little lady couldn't hear at what could have been her final birthday celebration, so I agreed to the terms.

Another patient suffering with a severe hearing loss desperately needed hearing aids to maintain his employment. However, his credit rating was poor because his ex-wife cleaned out their savings and overextended their credit cards before she ran off with the mailman. At least that was the story he told. Although the man was down on his luck, he guaranteed me that he would pay his balance within three months if I would find it in my heart to help him.

Well, following the birthday party, the aged woman returned the aids for credit because she only wanted to hear for her party, and what portion of the balance for the man that was down on his luck did I collect? Zip, zilch, zero. I spent a lot of time with these two folks that I wasn't reimbursed for not to mention the acquisition of the man's hearing aids. Many people will have a story and a reason not to pay *today*, but the fact is it takes money to run a business. Patients will give every imaginable and sometimes unimaginable reason not to pay their balance, but you have to find a comfortable way to say, "This is your balance. How would you like to take care of that today?" Financial analysts report that poor cash flow is the number one killer of small businesses.

A written policy sets guidelines regarding the handling of payments and assures that all patients are treated fairly and equitably. When patients balk at paying, it will be easy to say, "This is our collection policy. Unless you have made other arrangements with Dr. _____, I will need a 50% deposit today. How would you like to handle that? We accept cash, checks, and credit cards." In many practices, collections are managed by a staff member in an effort to avoid negative experiences that could interfere with the doctor/patient relationship.

Most hearing health care practices can't afford to act as a bank for its patients. If insurance doesn't pay for a service or device, make it clear to patients when they schedule appointments that they will be required to pay for services when they are rendered, and remind them of the anticipated fee when confirming their appointment. In the case of hearing aids, ask for half down when the aids are ordered and the remainder on delivery of the aids. You may even consider offering a small discount when a patient pays in full with cash or check at the time the order is placed. Make paying convenient by accepting cash, checks, and credit and debit cards, and consider offering a finance program. By accepting all forms of payment, you can eliminate most excuses for not paying at the time of service. As a rule of thumb, accounts receivable should never exceed one month's average gross revenue.

Statements should be sent regularly to patients who have a balance. It is a good idea to send statements when you are waiting to receive insurance monies to keep patients informed of what is happening with their accounts so they won't be surprised if they get a bill months later when their insurance pays less than expected. When planning your cash flow, always account for the fact that it usually takes people longer to pay than you expect.

When all else fails, it may be necessary to send past due accounts to collections. Be prepared to initiate collection proceedings for patients who refuse to pay their balances within a reasonable amount of time. Your options include hiring a collections agency or, for larger balances, filing a case in small claims court. A colleague of mine recently asked how I handle patients who refuse to pay their balance. It's simple. I will no longer see them. Personally, I would rather do something worthwhile, like work on my marketing plan, or go shoe shopping, than invest more time in someone who refuses to "show me the money."

Accounts Receivable Procedures

Charges entered at front desk when patient checks out following appointment.

The AR specialist reviews HCFA billing report and to bills insurance charges. The goal is to bill insurance charges within 48 hours of visit.

The AR specialist will conduct a review of all accounts receivables on the 7th and the 21st of each month. The AR specialist will prepare two reports for all outstanding invoices, with notes by the 21st of each month. This contains one report for insurance and one report for private pay. The reports will be sent to PHS COO.

<u>Statement processing for both insurance and private pay:</u>

1. The AR specialist will send statement to patient for remaining balance after insurance payment is posted.

2. Statements are sent to patients with any and all outstanding balances by 5th of the month—unless they have received a statement within the last two weeks.

3. If patient does not respond with payment by 1st of following month after patient is contacted, a second statement should be sent with note, "Please remit balance by end of month."

4. If patient does not respond with payment by 15th of month after second statement is mailed, the AR specialist contacts patient.

5. If patient does not respond following receipt of second statement, a third and final statement will be sent that states, "If your balance is not paid in full by end of the month, your balance will be sent to collections."

6. If payment is not received by the end of the month following the third and final statement, information is given to PHS COO and patient's balance is sent to collections.

<u>Insurance companies outstanding balances:</u>

Companies who have outstanding balances to us will be called <u>at least once per month</u> to update status of claims, and this information will be included in monthly AR report. If payment is not received within reasonable amount of time (45 days), a phone call will be extended to insurance company to see if the claim is pending or should be rebilled.

No write-offs of the above without approval from PHS COO.

Goal—Total of AR—less than_____ (excludes 0–30 days billed
to insurance)
   Total of AR—over 90 days—less than _____

Total AR should not exceed one month of total gross revenue.

Third Party Administrators (TPAs)— Friend or Foe?

The growth of TPAs in the hearing aid reimbursement process
has brought new challenges to hearing health care. These programs are being offered by traditional commercial payers and
their subsidiaries. Many of us are threatened with losing significant numbers of patients unless we agree to participate. Should
we or shouldn't we? When considering this dilemma, it comes
to mind that the only way to know for sure is to have a good
handle on the status of the business. I have preached the **need
for tracking** for years, and it's more necessary than ever in
these tenuous times. We may all *think* we know how much our
businesses could be affected by these TPAs, but we *really don't
know for sure* unless we have the numbers to back up those feelings. The consequences of saying "Yes" or "No" could negatively
impact the business forever.

In order to make informed decisions regarding whether to
participate with these programs, it's necessary to calculate the
break-even hourly rate for the practice, and this rate should
include desired profitability. This will determine how much revenue needs to be generated each and every hour for the business
to break even. A business can't stay alive if reimbursement isn't
equal to or greater than the break-even hourly rate. If we accept
reimbursement that is lower than the break-even point, we will
find ourselves working harder for the same, or less, money.
That doesn't seem like much fun to me. Being busy isn't better
unless it's producing greater profitability for the business. Make
certain to understand the type of contract you are signing. Is it

discounted fee-for-service? Can you afford to provide the mandated services for the agreed reimbursement? Definitely clarify covered and noncovered services and products, and whether the payer allows for upgrades beyond covered services, as one's ability to upgrade beyond the covered service amount can be key for acceptable reimbursement, especially for those who dispense hearing aids. Also check the terms for reimbursement. It is not uncommon for third-party payer contracts to delay reimbursement for 45 to 60 days post service. You have to make certain that you have the cash flow to cover delayed reimbursement if you are used to getting paid when services are rendered.

If you have an existing business, perhaps the answer to the question of participating with TPAs is not in participating, but rather in doing a better job and staying more connected with current patients, thus creating more opportunities for them to hear well. My practice currently does not participate with the majority of these programs, and we continue to do well, but we do have to hustle to make up for the business that we have lost by not participating. We have increased marketing efforts in an attempt to attract new business, but that is expensive. We have also seen some success in working with local companies to become the preferred providers for their employees and their families. When backed into a corner, it's possible to find new avenues for business that you may not have discovered if it wasn't essential for business growth. The decision is a business decision but with the growing number of these programs, my practice may be forced to participate with these programs.

So, what's the right answer to participating with TPAs? Only you can determine what is right for your business, but the only real way to make the right decision is to know your numbers!

9

Business Essentials

I was chatting with a colleague recently who shared that she was struggling with her business. Schedules were full and everyone seemed to have more work to do than time to do it, and yet despite all the activity, profitability was declining. She was investigating ways to attract new patients, and contemplating adding more staff to handle the increased workload. If all else failed, the frustrated business owner was convinced that opening an additional location would solve all her problems. As our discussion continued, it became obvious that she was convinced that more patients would be the answer to her problems. This made me wonder, "When is more not better?" Passing thoughts as I answered myself included: more weight when the pants don't fit; more alcohol when you have already had one too many; more men if you are already married to one, or more offices if they add expenses, extra work, and not additional profit. As my mind shifted from the amusing to the more serious topic of business, a few ideas came to mind.

Patients who come for free screenings or free trials and never purchase anything are not adding to the bottom line of a business. Lots of people will say yes to something that is advertised as free, but how many really want to improve their hearing? It's unfortunate but many patients are not really committed unless they have something invested. When considering whether to do anything for free, remember that time is money and any time invested in someone who really isn't interested in improving their hearing costs the business money.

Bundling services into the price of a hearing aid is common practice for many in this industry. Because a business really can't afford to see patients for free, it's essential to determine how many times the average patient will be seen during the use of the hearing aid, and to build adequate dollars into the initial price to cover the cost of those visits. For those who bundle services into the price of hearing aids, it may be beneficial to have a detailed breakdown available for patients as to what is included in the price, and what those services would cost if the fees were not bundled into the price of the aids. Price is what you pay and value is what you get. If a business model includes a bundled service plan, then it's important to let patients know the value of the services they will be receiving that are included in the plan. The services in a bundled plan are not free because patients are paying up front for the services so they don't have to pay as they go. Although bundling is not appropriate for every business, some patients prefer a bundled service plan.

If a business is growing, it will reach a point when the owner can no longer manage all the required tasks. When you are unable to serve patient's needs in a timely manner, or if patients are going to your competitor because you are too busy to see them, it is time to think about adding an employee. At this point, the real question is what type of staff will best serve the business needs: professional or support staff? Never add staff simply because an employee complains of being too busy. "Busyness" does not equal productivity. An employee's activity level may not be a reflection of their value to the business. For most organizations, employees represent not only their main asset, but also their largest investment. Making effective use of that investment by ensuring reasonable productivity is fundamental. Realistic goals and objectives are necessary to maintain focus and to insure productivity. Businesses change, and policies and procedures must reflect those changes. Therefore, employers should periodically assess job descriptions to ensure that current procedures match the present needs of the business. Reviews of employee performance should take place at least once a year.

Growth and expansion require careful planning. The decision to expand must be a result of thoughtful consideration of various factors, including financial, logistical, practical, and even the owner's emotional readiness. According to the Small Business Association, the rule of thumb is that a business should only expand when there are untapped opportunities that can benefit the business. For instance, if new patients are having to wait more than a week to get into the schedule, it is time to assess how appointments are scheduled and what types of tasks are included. Professionals should be spending most of their time diagnosing hearing abilities, solving problems when patients are not hearing well, and on activities that generate revenue for the business. If a professional's schedule is filled with nonrevenue-generating activities, it's time to do a time study to determine what activities that do not require the education and expertise of the professional can be delegated to support staff. It's important to determine what it costs the business for every hour of professional time. An example of how to calculate the cost follows, and this example is based upon the average number of hours a full-time professional works per year, and a hearing health care practice that generates $300,000 of gross revenue per year (Figure 9–1).

Expanding operations does not always mean more profit. The fact is a business may be doing more volume by adding a second or third location, and the owner will definitely be working harder, but with additional overhead, profitability may not improve, and, in fact, may even decline during the initial phase of expansion. It's not a good idea to open another location as a reaction to what the competition is doing.

Owning and operating multiple locations isn't for everyone. Some practice owners are content operating a single location and being the sole service provider, while others may want to create a chain of hearing health care organizations. The average

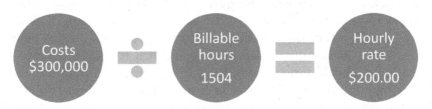

Figure 9–1. High water hides the stumps.

hearing health care practice in the United States consists of a single location with one service provider and one support staff. If run properly, this type of practice can produce a very respectable income for the owner.

Perhaps the answer is not in having more patients but in doing a better job with current patients, making certain to maintain contact by scheduling regular visits. However, every visit does not necessarily need to be handled by the professional. Appointments for routine hearing aid cleanings can be handled by support staff, as long as state licensure laws allow it. The annual assessments of aided performance should be scheduled with professionals to ensure that every opportunity is taken to help patients have the best hearing possible. Only you can determine what is right for your business. But when is more better? The only time I am certain of the answer to that question is when it comes to shoes. In that case, more is definitely better.

Details that Matter

Early one morning on a recent vacation, I dashed down to the local Starbucks to get some much-needed coffee for my husband and me. Our hotel was enormous with several wings on each floor. When I returned with the giant cups of java, I noticed the door to the room was half-open. I burst in announcing my arrival and quickly realized the half-clothed, rather large man coming forward was definitely not my husband. I caught a glimpse of the stunned look on his face and turned to run, spilling coffee all over his room on my exit.

Believe it or not, this wasn't the first time I have found myself in such a predicament. As I attempted to explain my seemingly bad luck to my husband, he gently suggested that these recurring events happen because I am always in a hurry and don't pay enough attention to details. Of course, I am in a hurry! I run a business. Although I would never admit it to him, I knew he was right. This led me to wonder if I overlook details in life, am I paying enough attention to details in business. Business owners wear multiple hats. We manage employees, develop marketing plans and budgets, pay bills, and monitor referral sources—not to mention that we see patients and fit in the demands of family and social responsibilities. It is easy to understand how a few details can get overlooked. However, details can be critical to the long-term success of a business.

Although discussing the impact of the current economy on the state of his long-time business, a business consultant that I had hired made a comment that really hit home with me, "High water hides the stumps." I immediately knew what he was referring to. Past years have been kind to hearing health care practices. Demand for the services we provide and the products we dispense has been high and our profit margins have been good. Although we are still in a fabulous profession with bright hopes for business in the future, hearing health care is facing challenges in the form of reduced reimbursement, an onslaught of third party administrators, and increased competition, just to name a few. These challenges necessitate the need to run a "lean and mean" business. When business is thriving, it is easy to overlook or ignore costs that may be out of line, but when times get tough, it becomes essential to search for ways to reduce as many costs as possible. The cost of doing business changes frequently and prices must reflect those changes. I have glanced at an invoice and overlooked a slight increase in shipping or a minor charge for an accessory, but a few small increases can translate to a major reduction in profitability. Monitoring profit and loss on a monthly basis will assist in keeping a handle on the cost of operating and maintaining a practice. A good place to start in assessing profit and loss is to consider the cost of the space you occupy. If you are purchasing the building in which you reside, reduced interest rates may represent a significant savings in mortgage payments. If you are renting, perhaps you could negotiate a discount in price per square footage, or in the triple-net costs you may be paying. Costs for telephone and Internet services can vary greatly by provider. I experienced an incident recently when I called a cable company to cancel my services because the costs had become what I felt to be exorbitant, and they offered me a much lower rate without my even asking for one. No cost is too low to investigate and negotiation is always an option. Check to see how much you are spending on little-used Yellow Page ads and assess how many of your patients actually choose your office because of the Yellow Pages. Many consumers use Internet directories so you may be able to cut spending without affecting business. Regularly investigate shipping charges, as many suppliers fail to notify businesses of small increases. Consider combining shipments or charging patients when superfast service is requested. Don't use snail mail unless necessary, and evaluate which items can be e-mailed or sent via text message. Many seniors are very tech savvy and would prefer texts over phone calls or e-mails, so ask your patients how they would like to receive information from you.

One of the questions I hear colleagues express is that they really don't know if their business is doing well. What is typical gross revenue and net profit for a practice? The question is a good one. How does one know if their practice is actually doing well and could or should the business be doing better? The answer is a personal one. If you are generating a profit over and above expenses and you are making a wage that is appropriate for your education and the time you are investing, then that is success! Don't let other people's goals drive your business. Set your own and then watch and manage the numbers so your business is producing the result that you want (Figure 9–2).

Major Expenses

The average hearing health care practice has two major expenses —the cost of goods and the cost of employees. In most practices, the biggest expense is the cost of goods sold (COGS), which, in most cases, are hearing aids. If your COGS is more than 35%, investigate whether your prices need to be increased and if necessary, contact your suppliers and attempt to renegotiate prices, or if you are in a network or buying group, perhaps it is time to determine if they are adding value or if you should "go it alone." I will contend that if you are buying over 10 aids a month from one supplier you probably can negotiate a better price by being independent. Also, consider the number of manufacturers you

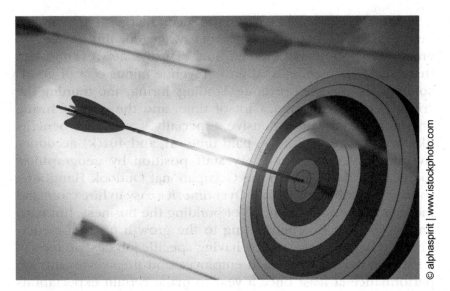

© alphaspirit | www.istockphoto.com

Figure 9–2. Go for the goals!

are using, as the more you buy, the better price you can usually negotiate. If a price reduction is not possible, try to negotiate free shipping, extended warranties, or extra receivers at no charge, or simply investigate other suppliers and their pricing. Are you examining invoices closely to make sure pricing hasn't changed, or that you are getting charged for items that you aren't charging your patients for? It is easy to lose track of small price increases in a busy practice, and small increases can really cut into profits.

It should go without saying that every business owner should periodically review relationships with vendors and suppliers to make certain that they are offering competitive prices and delivering quality service. In most hearing health care businesses, manufacturing partners are a very important part of the business. However, it's wise to keep a close eye on invoices to make certain that there haven't been any major price increases, and that you are paying a fair price for products. This investigation can also serve as a good way to review the prices you are charging patients to make sure your margins are in line with the cost of doing business.

Employee costs are usually the second largest expense in a business. My CPA suggests that total wages for the owner and employees should not exceed 30% of gross net revenue and that can be defined as total gross revenue minus cost of goods sold equals gross net revenue. Finding, hiring, and training the "right person" can take a lot of time, and the cost of hiring an employee can be expensive, especially if you offer benefits like health care insurance, paid time off, and 401(k) accounts. Average pay scales for every staff position by geographical location can be found in the Occupational Outlook Handbook (https://www.bls.gov/ooh/). Over time, it's easy to hire more and more employees in the hope of building the business, but each employee must be contributing to the growth of the practice. This can only be assessed by having specific job descriptions of what is expected from each employee and then reviewing job performance at least once a year to make certain expectations are being met.

Making a concerted effort to retain your current patient base is good for business. Do you stay in touch and schedule regular visits? Although staying in touch with your patient base may take some time, it will be worth it. Some patients leave an audiology practice because they relocate or pass away, but the majority of them leave because of a perceived attitude of indifference. Many hearing health care providers concentrate the preponderance of their resources and energy on searching for new patients, while often ignoring the opportunities that exist with current ones. Because the cost for acquiring a new patient is almost five times more than that of retaining a current patient, it's critical to the profitability of a practice to maintain a relationship with a patient for as long as you can, or preferably, forever.

Marketing can be a conundrum for most business owners. What will work? What won't work, and how much will you have to spend to find out? Marketing is important because you need it to grow a business, but it can be a huge endeavor and one that's difficult to fit into a schedule when you are also seeing patients and running the business. Marketing costs can get out of control very quickly. There are innumerable mediums to place your message, so it's key to measure and monitor what you are getting from every dollar you spend. As I mentioned earlier, if you are still paying for Yellow Page advertising you probably just need to STOP. Many consumers use Internet directories, but traditional Yellow Page advertising is *Out* and social media is *In*. It's possible to reach a large audience with Facebook and other social mediums for a much smaller cost than traditional outreach marketing.

One of the fastest ways to get into a cash flow crisis is to provide goods and services to slow-paying customers, and that includes insurance companies. If payment gets too slow, it may be necessary to discontinue participation with certain third-party payers. Although this may seem like a drastic move, if you aren't getting paid or if you are providing services at dramatically reduced rates, it may be costing the business more than it is benefiting it. It's OK not to participate with *every* discount or third-party administrator program. If the fees aren't paying for your time, then it may not be worth participating. An option to improve cash flow is to offer financing or small incentives (1% to 2%) when patients pay in full by cash or check at the time of order. You can't give an additional discount if someone is paying with a credit card because you are already paying a fee to the credit card company. Shop around for credit card rates and make sure you are getting the best possible rate.

Some of the best advice I ever received was from my accountant many years ago. "Get your money up front. You don't have the money of a bank so don't try to act like one." Wise words of wisdom that have served me well over the years. When patients ask if they have to pay now, I simply say, "Yes. Payment is expected when services are rendered." Period. No exceptions.

It's been discussed earlier that many hearing health care practices that dispense hearing aids bundle and include a service package in the cost. If you provide care to a patient and the cost wasn't bundled and covered up front at the time of purchase, you must charge the patient for your time. The number of Internet discount programs and direct-to-consumer sales are increasing exponentially, and more third-party payers are only paying for a small number of follow-up visits. A business cannot afford to provide services and not get paid for them. You may consider offering comprehensive service programs if the plans you offer to patients do not bundle services into the cost of hearing enhancement. You can also offer extended warranty or service programs to patients once the original plan expires. This is a great way to keep patients connected to you and your practice. Hearing aids are an investment and patients are often willing to protect that investment, especially if the professional they trust feels it will benefit them.

Patient satisfaction is an important predictor of patient retention, and retention is becoming more and more critical to the success of a business. It is helpful to send satisfaction surveys to patients three to five months after they purchase new hearing aids. And pay attention to their answers. Also, ask every patient who visits your office how they are doing and if she or he is happy with your services. You may be surprised at the answers!

When business is good and things are going smoothly, it's easy to take referral sources for granted. It's also easy to make the mistake of spending too much time courting referrals from sources that will never make a referral to you. The most common mistake I see practitioners make is treating all their contacts as if they were sources of referrals. It's ineffective because it doesn't get you the results you want. For instance, an otolaryngologist that has an audiology department will probably never refer to an outside source so don't spend time courting those referrals. You won't be able to convince every family practice doctor or every pediatrician to refer to you, so spend your time on the ones that have already sent you patients. When you value a referral source, make sure to cultivate the relationship by visiting the office every month. Promote regular communication, and let that person know you value and appreciate their referrals.

10

Focus on Possibilities

While vacationing in Arizona recently, my friend convinced me to start my day with an invigorating walk. He assured me he knew a great route that wouldn't be too tough. After we trekked for about a mile, I was confronted with a very long road that rose steeply into the mountains. "You didn't say we were climbing a mountain," I protested. As we walked up the steep incline for what seemed to me hours, my attitude deteriorated with every step. This wasn't exactly how I wanted to start my vacation. After almost 45 minutes and lots of grumbling, I made it to the top and vowed to myself that this was the last walk I would take with that friend.

The next day, my friend suggested we conquer that same mountain again. "Why would I want to do that?" I thought. However, not one to back down from a challenge, I gathered my energy and set out for the long, arduous hike. This time I decided I would embrace the opportunity to burn some calories and start my day in a healthy way. As the journey progressed, I noticed that I wasn't as out of breath and it didn't seem nearly as difficult as the previous day. I was actually having fun! When the walk ended, I realized the only thing that had changed from the previous day was my attitude. If my attitude affected my performance on that walk, could my attitude be affecting my performance at work? One thing I have learned over the many years of owning and working in my business is . . .

Attitude is Everything

If you believe it will be a good day, then it is, but if you walk into the practice and feel it's going to be a bad day, that prediction will also come true! All you have to do is listen to a news report to start getting a bad attitude. Those pessimistic newscasters make me feel like Chicken Little. After watching the morning news, I am certain that the sky is falling and I begin living cautiously and staying awake nights worrying about the economy and the future of my business. Yet, my worrying doesn't change anything. Although I understand that the economy is not what it was and this may affect my practice, I also know that despite the economic downturn, people still want and need to hear better.

There is much evidence that people who think positively are more successful than those who think negatively. Norman Vincent Peale, the original positive thinker and author of *The Power of Positive Thinking* said, *Change Your Thoughts and You Can Change Your Life*. Anthony Robbins, a motivational guru, commands huge fees to present his high-energy lectures on the subject. I also have my own stories that reinforce the effects of positive thinking. There is a constant battle in our minds between positive and negative thoughts, and the more negative things we listen to, the greater our chance of being controlled by negativity. Whereas it is important to know what's happening in the world, we don't need 24/7 news to stay informed. Thirty minutes twice a day may be ample time to stay in touch. The more we give into negative thoughts, the more negative we become. Negative thinking can destroy our dreams, so if we are going to reach our potential, we must guard against negative thinking and anything that promotes negativity. We must purposely build positive energy within ourselves. I have several favorite books on positive thinking and I start every day by reading key passages that inspire me. My favorite is *The Wealthy Spirit: Daily Affirmation for Financial Stress Reduction* by Chellie Campbell. She points out that most people look to outside factors to bring them happiness, and are ultimately disappointed when their dreams don't turn out the way they had planned or expected. Campbell's book is composed of a series of daily affirmations that focus on the reader's internal strength and capacity for change. It's a must read in my life (Figure 10–1).

Making a conscious decision to take action is one of the defining differences between people who achieve great things and those who settle for mediocrity. No one said being a success is easy, but it won't happen unless we make the conscious decision to succeed. I encourage everyone to take a few minutes to write down five goals for their life and then look and review them at least once a month. Everything we have (or don't have) in life is a result of the actions we take. Making a commitment to take action to achieve your goals is like putting a car in gear. It's the first step toward reaching a destination. Decide what you

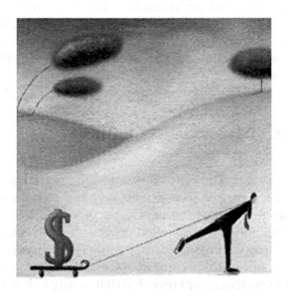

The Wealthy Spirit

Daily Affirmations for Financial Stress Reduction

Chellie Campbell

Copyrighted Material

Figure 10–1. My favorite book.

want in life, develop a plan, and then consciously go after it and don't stop until you can mark the goal as "*I did it!*"

Don't let the state of the economy or some pundit's predictions become the driving force of your business. Sure, everyone faces adversity in life, but successful people believe they can overcome those hardships and reach their goals. Focus on the outcomes you want instead of the outcomes you fear, and don't hesitate to think big. Nelson Mandela said, "There is no passion in living small and in settling for a life that is less than what you are capable of living." I feel fortunate to be in a great profession that offers enormous potential in both good and lean economic times. Achieving starts with believing. You must have faith that you can and WILL accomplish your goals. Start today and focus on the positive, reach for your goals, and never accept the idea that there is a limit to how far you can go. By the way, remember the story I started this chapter with? With my friend's encouragement, I climbed that mountain twice on the last day of my vacation!

Embrace Necessary Change

There is a saying, "The only constant in life is change." So if this is true, why are people so resistant? Perhaps it's because they are afraid. Change can cause careers to become obsolete, employees may lose their jobs, or automated processes may replace employees in a company. In many cases, people resist change because it moves them out of their comfort zones into unfamiliar territory. A study at livescience.com revealed that nearly half of all patients diagnosed with early stage lung cancer went back to smoking after less than a year, so even the threat of death wasn't enough to force people to change!

While we are very fortunate in this profession that despite the many challenges that we are facing, the future continues to look bright, we are certainly in need of some change. Technology is moving fast, but unfortunately, many of our clinical protocols need modification and some practitioners are not keeping pace with the ever-changing industry. Not only is wireless technology revolutionizing the products and subsequent benefits we can offer our patients, electronic media is transforming the way the world communicates. A recent article purported that online hearing testing and in-home hearing aid fitting was just as reliable and valid as what we do in our offices. So, if change is inevitable, what changes can hearing health care professionals embrace to keep pace with the ever-changing world? Certainly, it is prudent to start automating as many processes as possible, and electronic records are a mandate and no longer just an option.

Automation reduces error and the need for continuous manual review of records. By adopting electronic medical records, processes such as insurance billing can be streamlined. Digitizing and automating the billing process enables faster collections, fewer denials, and more consistent flow of revenue. Most practice management software includes an automated billing module.

Most patients today have access to e-mail and are familiar with the internet. Find a resource to send automated email or text messages to your patients whenever you have news or information to share. When a patient doesn't have access to e-mail, most office management software has the potential to send automated letters. If you are the revenue generator in your practice, your time should be spent with patients, not on addressing envelopes.

The patient experience has become the new professional battleground in health care and hearing health care is no exception. Patients can go anywhere, and I do mean anywhere, to obtain hearing health care services. I have read that patient satisfaction in this industry is more dependent on how patients are treated than by how well they hear. Because satisfied patients are more likely to spread positive word of mouth about the benefits of better hearing, catering to the patient experience is a necessity.

There is evidence in the industry that nearly one-third of hearing aids have not been properly fit and the resultant settings are not providing optimal gain and benefit for the patient. Several recent studies have shown that hearing health care professionals and the best practices employed by these professionals play a significant role in patients' success. It is simply unacceptable to let a real ear machine become anything more than a dust collector, and recorded speech testing should be the norm. The majority of patients experience difficulty hearing in background noise, so speech in noise testing is essential for giving patients realistic expectations for hearing aid use. And, of course, giving patients the experience of listening to hearing aids in your office while having noise play in the background is a good start for establishing those expectations.

There is a strong relationship between quality hearing health care, benefit, and quality of life improvements. Benefits always outweigh price in this industry, so instead of lowering prices, adhere to a best practices protocol consisting of a comprehensive test battery, including measures of loudness discomfort, speech-in-noise testing, and complete real-ear measurements to ensure that patients are deriving optimal benefit from their hearing aids.

Certainly, we have the means to provide more appropriate fittings, but the deterrent may be time itself. This is not surprising because the average practitioner is not only seeing patients, but also burdened with cumbersome paperwork required by third-party payers and the many tasks involved in running a business. Obviously, one person can't do everything successfully. The change we need may be using assistants to perform the tasks that do not require the education and expertise of a hearing health care professional. The use of audiology assistants has been endorsed by every professional organization for the past forty-five years and yet the practice is only embraced in less than 50% of audiology employment settings.

Return for credit rates as measured by manufacturers, including exchanges, have hovered around 20% to 25%. Returns for credit are extremely detrimental to a business. Not only have we lost a patient when someone returns their hearing aids, but there is another person in the community spreading the word that hearing aids don't work! Set a goal to reduce returns for credit to less than 2%. We set that goal and our returns for credit are less than 2% of all sales. We simply won't settle for anything less. This 2% is simply returns for credit and does not include exchanges but we keep those to a minimum.

Make certain to perform the necessary outcome tests to insure that patients are hearing as well as possible before they leave with the hearing aids. This includes performing aided testing for an annual evaluation. When I visit my optometrist, he doesn't just ask me how well I am seeing, he tests how well I am seeing with my present prescription. We should be doing the same with our patients. If a patient has poor speech in noise ability, recommend a rehabilitation program or app for them to use at home to improve their ability to understand in noise or recommend an assistive device that may improve hearing In noise.

Although change is not easy for anyone, we can embrace it and let it transform our lives or we can fight it and let it be the bane of our daily existence. I look at change in the same way I look at disagreements with my husband. Sometimes it is easier to surrender than fight (Figure 10–2).

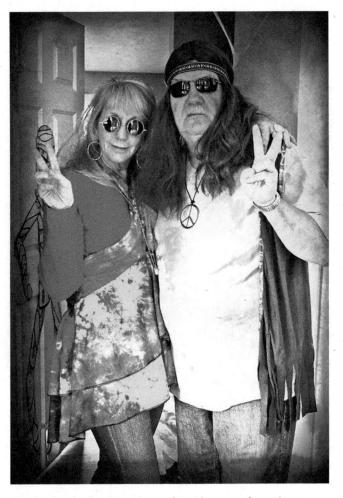

Figure 10–2. David and me after 40 years of marriage.

11
Developing an Exit Strategy

After a particularly frustrating month, I advised my financial planner to "up" the stakes so I could retire earlier than originally planned. Although I probably won't, there are days when you want to slam the door, walk away, and never look back. The new plan came in a few days and all I could say was, "WOW. That's not going to happen!" Even though I felt I was on track for retirement, it is unbelievable how much money it will take to maintain my present lifestyle for what may be another 40 years!

The truth is that many business owners don't plan soon enough. Although your practice may provide a very nice living, it also must provide enough excess cash to invest so you can one day retire and live as comfortably as you did when you were working. This will definitely require a strategy years in the making that is periodically reevaluated to make certain you stay on track.

One favorite exit strategy of some business owners is simply to bleed the company dry on a daily basis. I don't mean run it in the red; I mean pay yourself a nice salary and reward yourself with frequent dividends so that at the end of the year, there is nothing left. This type of strategy is sometimes called "Lifestyle Company." Rather than reinvesting money in growing your business, in lifestyle companies, you keep things small, take out a comfortable chunk, and simply live on the income.

Another exit strategy is simply to call it quits, close the business' doors, and walk away. Certainly we have all had days when we wanted to do just that, and this is a possibility as long as you have saved or invested enough money to live off for the rest of your life and are not counting on the value of your business to fund your retirement. Just make sure that you have had a professional assess how much money this will take, as you may be very surprised.

The easiest strategy may be passing ownership to another hearing health care professional, a person who will preserve your legacy and continue to serve your patients. An obvious choice for this rite of passage may be an employee who understands the business or one who is hired intentionally to assume ownership of the business. The fictional Willy Wonka handed off his chocolate empire to a little boy who was a loyal Wonka customer, someone who was chosen with great care through a selection process designed to weed out all but the most dedicated Wonka devotees. The biggest problem may be finding someone who has the money to buy the business. Often, in this kind of strategy, the seller finances all or part of the sale and lets the buyer pay it off over time. It can be a win-win for everyone involved, but there is also some risk involved. How will the owner pay you back if business deteriorates and there isn't adequate cash to make the payments?

Acquisition is another type of exit strategy. In past years, there has been a trend of manufacturers acquiring private practices to guarantee distribution of their products. In an acquisition, the owner and proposed buyer negotiate a price and that price is usually based on the "value" of the practice. There are a many ways to value a business. There's no one right way, though you could probably come up with several wrong ones. Ultimately, the business is worth whatever you think it's worth, based on the criteria you set forth, but the trick is finding someone who will pay you what you think the business is worth.

You can start by looking at the value of the business's assets. What does the business own? What equipment and how old is the equipment? How much inventory in stock? What is the total of the accounts receivable? After all, you'd have to buy all the same stuff if you were starting a practice from scratch, so the business is worth at least the replacement cost of these items.

A balance sheet can give a good indication of the value of the company's assets.

Another approach is to look at the cash flow of the business. Revenue is the crudest approximation of a business's worth. If the business generates $300,000 gross revenue per year, you can think of it as a $300,000 revenue stream. Often, businesses are valued at one time their gross revenue or some multiple of net revenue.

Entrepreneurs live with the struggle of launching their own businesses and then keeping that business alive. One thing we often forget is that decisions made on day one can have huge implications down the road. You see, it's not enough to build a business worth a fortune. It's a good idea to make sure you have an exit strategy, a way to get the money back out after all the time and money that has been invested over the years.

12

Dr. Gyl's Tips for Success

There is no *one* thing that makes a business successful, but if you get stuck and wonder what to do next, here are some quick tips for success:

Limit Partnerships

Starting a business with a partner offers many benefits, not the least of which is having someone to share the responsibilities of running a business, but I have seen a few turn very sour without sufficient forethought and planning. It's essential that the details of the partnership are in writing and specific before the doors of the business open. Another important relationship to consider is the one with your manufacturing partners. It's been my experience that the fewer manufacturers you use, the better the relationship. The more eggs you put into one basket, the better the pricing, customer service, and the greater expertise you will hopefully have with the products. Some business owners maintain a relationship with a professional network and/or buying group. Although these groups can provide valuable input into how to run a successful business, there will come a time when you have learned all you can from them, and yet the relationship increases costs. I think of these groups as training wheels for a business—you learn what you can and then it's time to go it alone.

Continually Search for New Ways to Help Patients

Our industry is constantly changing and it is crucial to read current research and to be aware of the latest innovations. Anyone with a hearing loss is interested in hearing better. Don't assume that just because a person has a set of hearing aids that she or he wouldn't be willing to purchase new ones if it helped her or him to hear better. Know what's trending in the world of hearing health care. Stay abreast of the latest developments in technology and then tell patients about them. Strive to *Be the Best* at what you do.

Keep Employees Happy

I have read that most employees would rather have a few words of praise than a raise. Although I don't really get that, I know how important it is to appreciate your employees and to commend them when they do a great job. If your employees aren't enjoying their jobs and work environments, it will be difficult for them to put on a happy face for patients, and patients notice when employees are unhappy. I suggest at least monthly staff meetings. In fact, I know colleagues that have brief meetings every morning to pump up the staff and to talk through events of the day.

Create an Extraordinary Experience for Patients

The patient experience is the new competitive battleground in health care. Patients have higher expectations than ever before and they are quick to change providers if their expectations aren't met. The cost of acquiring a new customer far exceeds the cost of retaining an existing customer. Every organization should look for opportunities to enhance the patient experience and to make customer service the top priority. Good isn't good enough. You have to be a superstar when it comes to service and the patient experience.

Market. Market. Market.

You may think that you can hang up a shingle and patients will flock to your door but it's not true. If you want new patients and want to retain the patients you have, you have to market to them. Take every opportunity to tell patients and prospects about the awesome new technology and/or services that will help them live a better quality of life. Without marketing, your business may offer the best products or services in your industry, but none of your prospective patients would know about it. Marketing can be expensive and you can't afford to spend money on campaigns that aren't attracting new patients, so measure the outcome of every effort to know what's effective. Marketing a business successfully may require outside assistance from a consultant or from your manufacturing partners.

Collect Money Up Front

An accountant gave me some great advice years ago. "Don't try to be a bank for your customers. Get your money up front." Many people will ask if they can pay over time, or try to convince you to take installments. Just because they ask doesn't mean you have to comply with the request. That's what finance companies are for. I just read some research from our industry that indicates that people are more likely to purchase hearing aids when no- or low-interest options are offered. The program may cost you a little money up front, but sales may increase because of it.

Measure and Monitor Key Elements of Profitability

I feel like a broken record saying, "What gets measured gets monitored." It's been my experience that people who don't measure how well the business is doing are generally not doing as well as they think they are. I was recently discussing business with a young colleague and she contended that she had a 98% "Help Rate." Help Rate, also called a Close Rate in sales presentations, was defined in a previous chapter as the percentage of patients that have a hearing loss and need *help* in the form of hearing aids versus the percentage of patients that actually purchase hearing aids at the time of their visit. I was skeptical that a neophyte would actually be able to convince almost every patient she saw to purchase hearing aids because that is atypical of most hearing healthcare professionals. However, after she reviewed her tracking sheets, her contentions did not prove to be accurate. When I looked at her schedule for a day, she had six new patients and no sales. Hmmm, something wasn't adding up and the tracking sheets certainly did not support the numbers she had shared with me. This happens over and over again (to me as well). Numbers don't lie! If you don't do anything else, measure and monitor your Help Rate, return for credit, average selling price, and cost of goods sold. Tracking is the first step to turning your business from Fine to Fabulous.

Focus on Best Practices

You may remember a study that came out several years ago that showed that over one-third of fittings are inappropriate and result in hearing aids being under fit. Perhaps we need to consider how we spend our time during the fitting process. I know many colleagues spend the majority of time during the fitting of new hearing aids teaching a patient how to insert the aids, explaining the maintenance and care of the units and how to change the batteries, and then press the best fit icon in the manufacturer's software. Verifying and validating performance of the hearing aids and ensuring that the prescribed gain is appropriate, as well as determining that the patient is hearing as well as possible, and that she or he won't be overwhelmed with sound, are some of the most important things we do. Focusing on best practices, such as real ear measures, aided discrimination and speech in noise testing to name a few, is a way to separate ourselves from the Big Box competition. If time is the issue, consider having an assistant complete the hearing aid orientation, and you, as the professional, can spend your time validating the fitting and ensuring it's as good as it can be. If that's not possible, then schedule more time for the fitting. It will pay off in the end.

Concentrate on Helping More Patients

I find it appalling that most hearing health care professionals convince less than half the people that need help by way of hearing aids to actually purchase them. You may as well get used to typical objections from patients that their hearing is not bad enough, and hearing aids are expensive, because you will hear that every day. Don't run from objections, learn how to handle them. If you believe that your practice or organization is the BEST place for the hearing impaired to obtain help, then make a commitment to convince more patients to accept your advice to do something about their hearing loss. Don't settle for mediocrity.

Set a Goal for What You Want for You and Your Business

Goals drive success. However, I have discovered in conversations with colleagues that many of them haven't actually established specific goals for themselves personally or professionally, or if they have, the goals aren't documented or written down. Goals without a formal action plan are merely dreams that probably will never happen. *If you shoot for nothing, you will hit it every time!* Start now and write down at least two goals that you would like to accomplish this year, and then devise a simple action plan to make them happen.

Reward Yourself

Nothing is more frustrating than working your butt off and then not being able to pay yourself a decent salary. Collecting a salary may not be possible in the early days of a business, but the goal should be to collect a salary. I know many colleagues who just get the "leftovers" and that isn't very satisfying. I was impressed when a colleague shared that she had grown her practice and now employed 17 full-time employees, but further discussion revealed that she didn't have the remaining funds to pay herself. A wise businessman once told me that if I was taking money out of my salary to pay another employee, perhaps I didn't really need that employee. Sure, there will be lean times when you can't pay yourself, but then you need to figure out what's causing the lean times and determine a course of action to improve profitability. If you don't have a budget, it's easier to spend money on things you can do without.

Although it isn't easy to manage the myriad of duties required to run a successful practice, you can do it. There are days when I, as I am sure many of you can relate to, have more to do than I have time! Although many tasks are important, it is essential to concentrate on completing the ones that bring revenue to the practice, such as attracting new patients, and keeping current patients satisfied and hearing as well as possible. Just try to remember that YOU don't have to do EVERYTHING. Ask yourself every time you start a task whether it is essential that you do it or whether you could delegate that task to a support person. If the task isn't generating revenue or helping to maintain a relationship with your current patients, then perhaps you don't need to do it.

When you are committed to making your business a success, working hard should be a joy rather than a burden. Doing what you love really isn't work. I believe the key to success is to never look back and only look forward. Business, like life, doesn't always go the way you plan it.

> Expect the best, plan for the worst, and do what it takes to survive!

Although you should expect bumps on the road to success, a successful business owner simply can't allow him or herself to have thoughts of failure. You can count on making mistakes, but it's not the mistakes that matter. It's how you recover from them (Figure 12–1).

I have been fortunate to meet so many awesome people around the globe that have taught me so much, but some of the best pearls of wisdom I have gathered have been from my patients. I recall a

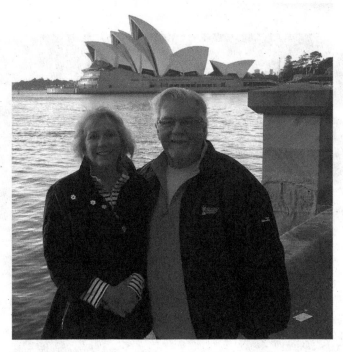

Figure 12–1. David and me in Australia.

patient that I fondly referred to as Uncle Henry. Henry was a very successful fruit farmer in my community—not really my uncle, but a much adored man by all who knew him. He came in one day for an appointment and shared that he was buying a large parcel of property to plant a new fruit orchard. I was pretty surprised by the idea considering, his advanced age of 96. I didn't think he would ever live to see the fruits of his labors. "It's not the outcome, my dear," Uncle Henry reminded me, "It's the vision." Don't let anything limit your vision. If you believe it, you can achieve it!

People always ask how I have created such a large practice in such a small town. They wonder how my business generates 10 times the revenue of the average practice when I live in a town of only 12,000 people. Yes, it's hard work, but it's not rocket science. It's just business and *Business is Business*, no matter where you practice. I've shared my business principles in this book and in my blogs at DrGyl.com, but I also offer an opportunity to show colleagues firsthand how to take their practices from *Fine to Fabulous* by hosting seminars at my

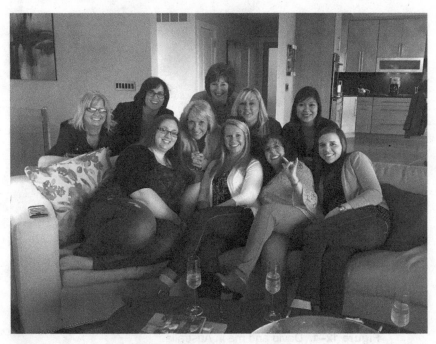

Figure 12–2. A group of attendees at a DrGyl Weekend.

practice in beautiful St. Joseph, Michigan. These are no ordinary seminars. I focus on hosting small, select groups, in which, along with some awesome and well-known colleagues, we present and share ideas for success. Then, I stay in touch with participants and mentor them to help them take their practices to a million-dollar level.

Participants have raved about my seminars and some come back multiple times. More information on my seminars can be found at DrGyl.com (Figure 12–2).

> "This woman is amazing and she helped me grow my business A LOT!!! Follow her, listen to her, attend her fabulous events in Michigan and you will reap the benefits! You won't be sorry!"
>
> —Gina Geissler, AuD, Hammond, Indiana
> Two-time seminar attendee

In Closing:
A Character Defining Moment

There is a lot of buzz today around the issue of women empowerment. I recall a time over thirty years ago when I had to deal with the issue. At the time, I was working one day a week doing diagnostics for two ENTs, and patients who needed hearing aids were referred to a hearing aid dispenser's office down the street. It didn't take long for me to realize that they were losing potential revenue from this arrangement, so I proposed that I would establish an audiology clinic and we would split the profits of testing and hearing aids, minus the cost of goods, 50/50. Keep in mind that this was many years ago and there were no regulations against such an arrangement. As an independent contractor, I paid my own taxes, received no paid time off, or any insurance benefits, and if I didn't generate revenue, I didn't get paid. It was my job to market the clinic, and when the business grew, I paid a receptionist out of my portion of the profits.

After three years of working my tail off and growing the practice, the ENTs informed me that I was making too much money and if I wanted to continue, it would be THEIR practice and I would be an employee for a salary much less than I had been making. When I challenged their offer and let them know that under no circumstances would I agree to such an arrangement, they reminded me that I was *just* an audiologist and they were ENTs. "How can you expect to make so much money when you are an audiologist?" they asked.

I consulted an attorney who definitely had some questions about the proposed contract. He wondered how I could have gotten myself involved in such an inequitable situation. "You need to learn to swim with the sharks without getting eaten," he offered. The ENTs were referring about 50% of the patients I was seeing, but the rest I had recruited myself. I had worked hard to grow the clinic and I knew that the ENT's portion of revenue was a significant amount of money for the small space I was occupying in their office, plus I was paying my own receptionist. I knew I needed to confront them, but I was nervous. I was a young female and they were middle-aged men with MD behind their names. Yet, I also knew that I couldn't respect myself if I stayed and let them walk all over me.

I met with the ENTs, reviewed the numbers, and explained why I believed that I was worth every penny I was making. Although they assured me that they liked me and thought I was doing a great job, it was very clear that they were not going to negotiate. "The salary we are offering is fair and much more than most audiologists make," they contended. The office was close to my house, the hours were great and I loved the patients, but I didn't even hesitate to say, "Thanks, but no thanks!" I think they thought I would change my mind, and they were quite surprised when I walked out and never looked back. I moved on, got a bank loan, and opened my own office. Besides marrying my husband, this has been the best decision that I ever made.

What I learned from that experience was instrumental to my success. It helped me see that I had the power to say, "No," and that I did not have to be held hostage to anyone or anything. It wasn't easy and I had to start over when I left but I have never wished I would have stayed because staying would have meant I was giving those ENTs power over my career and my life. The moral of this story is that we have to empower ourselves! We have to believe and remind ourselves that we have what it takes to succeed and no one can prevent us from reaching our goals.

The bottom line is we can't make decisions based upon what other people think. We have to do what is right for our lives regardless of whether another person likes that decision or not. What I've learned is that success is not measured by how much money I make, and my happiness does not come from pleasing other people. Happiness comes from inside. To me, empowerment happens when you realize that you, and only you, control your path and even though there may be bumps in the road, no one can derail you unless you let them. *We all have the power within us to be successful*. Don't settle for anything less.

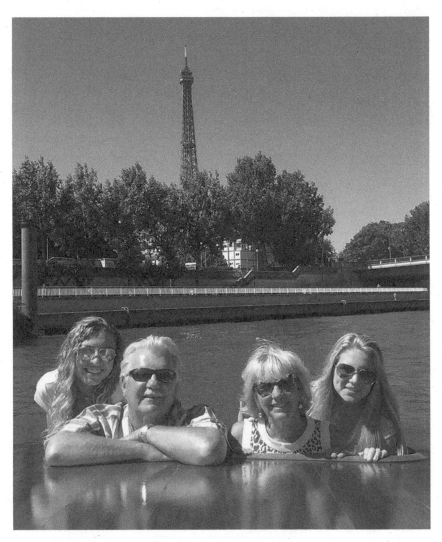

A recent trip to Paris, my favorite city.

Appendix:
Frequently Asked Questions

How Much Are Your Hearing Aids?

The cost of hearing aids varies based on what type of hearing loss you have. We have hearing aids and enhancement plans for ALL budgets! Let's get you scheduled and our professional can identify if you have a hearing loss and recommend a few options that fit within your budget. Do mornings or afternoons work best for you?

Our plans include not only the hearing aids, but als0 services and follow-up visits for one to three years, depending on the type of technology your purchase.

Does Insurance Pay for Hearing Aids?

Yes, depending on your insurance. We are willing to work with your insurance company to see what benefits they offer for hearing aids. Bring your insurance card when you come and we'll be happy to check your benefits at the time of your appointment.

Does Medicare Cover Hearing Aids?

Medicare does not typically pay for hearing aids. However, there are some medical supplement programs that may assist with paying for hearing aids. When you come in we will be happy to check your benefits.

Do You Accept Medicaid?

We do not accept Medicaid. We would be happy to provide you with a couple of names of practices that do accept Medicaid.

What's the Difference Between an Otolaryngologist, Audiologist, and Hearing Instrument Specialist?

Otolaryngologists and audiologists are both doctors; however, an otolaryngologist is an M.D. who specializes in surgery of the ear and nose, while an audiologist holds a clinical doctorate and specializes in hearing difficulties. A hearing instrument specialist specializes in hearing instrument technology and has met the minimum educational requirements of the state. Not all hearing instrument specialists have the same education. We can't speak to the training of others, however our HIS, Tony Meyer, has a Bachelors degree from MSU and continues to receive ongoing training and support from our two audiologists. All of our professionals stay up to date with the latest in hearing and hearing aid advancements.

Why Should I Choose You Instead of Another Company?

Choose any of our "Why Us" options:

- Our professionals know their stuff! With **years of experience** in the hearing wellness industry, our patients receive the best possible treatment and care.
- Our **world-class facility** is equipped with state-of-the-art equipment and the latest technology for evaluating your hearing abilities.
- PHS is the example for others. We set the **benchmark for practices** around the country in both patient care and patient satisfaction.

- We love what we do! We have a **passion** for serving people and helping patients improve their quality of life.
- We love to spoil our patients! We do so by **exceeding all expectations**.
- We are committed to **total patient satisfaction** and we will settle for nothing less.
- A visit to our office will be a **unique experience**, unlike any you've ever encountered before!
- You will receive the most **comprehensive testing**, allowing us to understand your unique level of hearing loss.
- **We care**, and we show that we do by being involved in the communities in which we live and work.
- We have **cookies**! Who doesn't love fresh baked cookies?!?

What Happens During the Hearing Evaluation Appointment?

The professional will check your ears for wax before taking you to the sound booth to perform the hearing evaluation. The assessment will consist of a series of tests that will measure your ability to hear beeps, words, and phrases. The professional needs you to bring your spouse/loved one along so they can use their voice during the testing process. The professional will share with you the results of the tests and any recommendations if you do have a hearing loss.

Do You Test for Hearing Loss in Children?

Yes, we can test children (ages 2 to under 18) for hearing loss. State law requires we perform a series of tests when evaluating the hearing of children. Depending on your insurance coverage, you may have out-of-pocket costs for the evaluation.

Index

Note: Page numbers in **bold** reference non-text material.